Oxford Handbook of
Mental Health Nursing

Edited by

Patrick Callaghan

Professor of Mental Health Nursing
University of Nottingham & Nottinghamshire
Healthcare NHS Trust

Helen Waldock

Health and Social Care
Advisory Service
London

OXFORD
UNIVERSITY PRESS

OXFORD
UNIVERSITY PRESS

Great Clarendon Street, Oxford OX2 6DP

Oxford University Press is a department of the University of Oxford.
It furthers the University's objective of excellence in research, scholarship,
and education by publishing worldwide in

Oxford New York

Auckland Cape Town Dar es Salaam Hong Kong Karachi
Kuala Lumpur Madrid Melbourne Mexico City Nairobi
New Delhi Shanghai Taipei Toronto

With offices in

Argentina Austria Brazil Chile Czech Republic France Greece
Guatemala Hungary Italy Japan Poland Portugal Singapore
South Korea Switzerland Thailand Turkey Ukraine Vietnam

Oxford is a registered trade mark of Oxford University Press
in the UK and in certain other countries

Published in the United States
by Oxford University Press Inc., New York

© Oxford University Press, 2006

British Library Cataloguing in Publication Data

Data available

Library of Congress Cataloging in Publication Data
Callaghan, Patrick.
Oxford handbook of mental health nursing/Patrick Callaghan and Helen Waldock.
p. ; cm. – (Oxford medical publications) (Oxford handbooks in nursing)
Includes bibliographical references and index.

1. Psychiatric nursing – Handbooks, manuals, etc. I. Waldock,
Helen. II. Title. III. Title: Handbook of mental health nursing. IV. Series. V. Series:
Oxford handbooks in nursing [DNLM: 1. Mental Disorders–nursing–Handbooks.
2. Mental Disorders–nursing–Nurses' Instruction. 3. Psychiatric Nursing–
methods–Handbooks. 4. Psychiatric Nursing–methods–Nurses' Instruction.
WY 49 C1560 2006]
RC440.C35 2006
616.89'0231–dc22   2006015488

Typeset by Newgen Imaging Systems (P) Ltd., Chennai, India
Printed in Italy
on acid-free paper by Legoprint S.p.A.

ISBN 978–0–19–856898–8 (Flexi.)

10 9 8 7 6 5 4 3 2

Foreword

This book, I believe, is destined to make a significant contribution to improving the quality of mental health care in the immediate future. Clients repeatedly relate that they wish to be cared for by health professionals who are kind, considerate and caring, but equally they desire personnel who are confident and knowledgeable. At no point in history has the need for informed carers been so pressing as it is today. Even those with the most passing interest in mental health services know that they are delivered within an increasingly complex arena. With the impending new legislation, new ways of working, and a greater emphasis on evidence-based interventions, this arena is set to become even more complex. Policies, guidelines, and frameworks have all played their part in endeavouring to improve services but there is one outstanding factor that is central to service improvement, namely, the presence of highly motivated, informed, and committed staff. Reviews of various professional training programmes have all concluded that information that remains in the minds of experts, academic institutions, and textbooks is of little use to those who deliver front-line services. For far too long it has been recognized that what these staff require is information that can be accessed instantly and in a manner and style that is both succinct and understandable. There are many excellent books on various aspects of mental health care, but this one is different. Its vast array of information is beyond the scope of specialist books.

In reading this book I am amazed at what has taken place with respect to the growth of information and the vast amount of scholarship that has been generated in mental health care during the course of my working life. In the early 1960s the amount of literature available to those undertaking psychiatric nurse training was sparse, amounting to no more than three or four assorted books. This book is testimony to what has happened since then and I am sure that readers will be impressed by the number of authors, largely mental health nurses, who have managed to present their material, on a wide range of topics, in a succinct and accessible way. On every page the reader will sense the enthusiasm of a young profession that is eager to seek knowledge and share it with others. I expect that readers will be impressed and humbled by the commitment of the authors in promoting the happiness and well-being of people with mental health problems and to removing obstacles that prevent clients from achieving everything that is within their power to do so.

The vision of the editors in bringing this book to fruition is to be commended. It deserves to become a high watershed in the history of mental health nursing scholarship and should be read by all mental health professionals, students, carers, clients, and those interested in mental health services. I was left with an overwhelming feeling of regret on reading this book that I am not about to start my career all over again. It is not a book to borrow, it is one you must own.

Professor Peter Nolan
Staffordshire University, Faculty of Health And Sciences

Preface

Currently, the mental health nursing textbooks available do not include anything in the format of a handy reference guide or a pocket-sized book with information that is readily accessible to the reader in a busy clinical setting. The aim of the *Oxford Handbook of Mental Health Nursing* is to provide practical, easily accessible, concise and up-to-date evidence-based guidelines covering all the essential elements of mental health nursing practice in one portable format.

Designed primarily for staff nurses and students, this book will assist anyone working with people living with mental health problems, and their families and carers, including junior doctors, medical students, occupational therapists, and social workers. It is envisaged that the more experienced clinician will be able to use sections for reference and as a resource for key facts.

This Handbook will enable readers to find relevant information quickly and will be small enough to carry in a mental health nurse's pocket or student's bag without taking up too much valuable space, and without the addition of unwanted weight.

We have arranged the contents in different sections for quick and easy access so as to provide up-to-date information about the essentials of mental health nursing practice in a user-friendly manner.

The book serves as a reference guide that supports nurses in everyday clinical decision-making and covers topics written by specialists in mental health nursing and related subjects that address the national mental health agenda.

It is our intention that the book be used by mental health nurses and others working across and within different areas of practice to improve the care of mental health service users, their carers, and families. We hope that the book enables mental health nurses to work in partnership with service users, their carers and other agencies, so that the users of mental health services recover from distressing mental health problems.

PC & HW

Acknowledgements

Mark Fenton—Editor, Database of Uncertainties about the Effects of Treatments (DUETs), Oxford.
Ms Jean Morrissey—Lecturer in Mental Health Nursing, Trinity College, Dublin.
Roselyn Musa BSc (Hons)—RNMH.

Contents

Detailed contents

2 **Essential mental health nursing skills**   59

4   Violence   **181**

5   Risk   **191**

6   Common mental disorders   **205**

Contributors

Dr Jane Alexander
Lecturer,
Department of Applied
Psychosocial Sciences,
City University, London

Ms Julie Attenborough
Senior Lecturer,
Department of Mental Health and
Learning Disability,
City University, London

Professor Len Bowers
Department of Mental Health and
Learning Disability,
City University, London

Mr Geoff Brennan
Nurse Consultant,
Prospect Park Hospital,
Tilehurst, Berkshire

Mr Dan Bressington
Lecturer,
Institute of Psychiatry,
Kings College, London

Dr Neil Brimblecombe
Director of Mental Health Nursing,
Department of Health & National
Institute of Mental Health in England

Mrs Jenny Cobb
Acting Head of Department,
Department of Mental Health and
Learning Disability,
City University, London

Mrs Tina Coldham
National Development
Consultant, Health and Social
Care Advisory Service, London

Mr Scott Durairaj
Diversity Lead. Mersey Care
NHS Trust

Ms Sarah Eales
Lecturer,
Department of Mental Health and
Learning Disability,
City University,
London

Mr Chris Flood
Lecturer,
Department of Mental Health
and Learning Disability,
City University, London

Mrs Cathe Gaskell
Deputy Chief Executive,
Nightingale House,
London

Dr Neil Gordon
Nurse Consultant,
Nottinghamshire NHS
Healthcare Trust

Professor Kevin Gournay MBE
Institute of Psychiatry,
Kings College,
London

Dr Richard Gray
Senior Lecturer,
Institute of Psychiatry,
Kings College,
London

Mr Paul Hammersly
Lecturer,
University of Manchester

Mr Ben Hannigan
Lecturer,
University of Cardiff

Dr Androulla Johnstone
Chief Executive,
Health and Social Care Advisory
Service

Dr Julia Jones
Senior Research Fellow,
Department of Mental Health and
Learning Disability,
City University, London

Ms Sarah Kendall
Clinical Research Fellow,
University of Manchester

Mr Ian Light (deceased)
Service User and Lecturer in
Mental Health and Social Care,
Department of Mental Health and
Learning Disability,
City University, London

Ms Mariya Limerick
Lecturer, School of Nursing,
University of Nottingham

Mr Peter Lindley
Sainsbury Centre for Mental
Health

Professor Karina Lovell
University of Manchester

Dr Eddie McCann
Lecturer, Primary Care
and Public Health Unit,
City University, London

Ms Shameen Mir
Chief Pharmacist,
East London and the City Mental
Health NHS Trust

Ms Soo Moore
Senior Lecturer,
Department of Mental Health and
Learning Disability,
City University, London

Ms Jean Morrissey
Lecturer,
Trinity College, Dublin

Ms Jan Murray
East London and the
City Mental Health NHS Trust

Ms Madeline O'Carroll
Lecturer, Department of Mental
Health and Learning Disability,
City University, London

Professor Sara Owen
University of Lincoln

Dr Peter Phillips
Lecturer,
Department of Mental Health
and Learning Disability,
City University, London

Dr Julie Repper
Reader in Mental Health,
University of Sheffield

Professor Dave Richards
University of York

Professor Paul Rogers
University of Glamorgan

Ms Rosemary Russell
Community Mental Health
Team Leader, Perth,
Western Australia

Professor Peter Ryan
Middlesex University

Mr Iain Ryrie
Assistant Director of Research,
Mental Health Foundation

Mrs Betsy Scott
Practice Education Manager,
East London and the
City Mental Health
NHS Trust

Dr Alan Simpson
Senior Research Fellow,
Department of Mental
Health and Learning Disability,
City University, London

Patricia McBride
Lecturer in Mental Health,
University of Paisley

Ms Phillippa Sully
Senior Lecturer,
Department of Applied
Psychosocial Sciences,
City University,
London

Ms Stephanie Tannis
Practice Education Manager,
East London and
the City Mental Health
NHS Trust

Mrs Johanna Turner
Performance Panel Coordinator
and Legal Advisor,
Newham PCT,
London

Ms Lynny Turner
Senior Lecturer,
Department of Mental Health and
Learning Disability,
City University, London

Mr Vince Turner
Community Psychiatric Nurse,
North East London Mental
Health Trust

Mr Malcolm Wandrag
Lecturer,
Department of Adult Nursing,
City University, London

Dr Richard Whittington
Reader in Mental Health,
University of Liverpool

Abbreviations

1°	Primary
2°	Secondary
↓	Decreased
↑	Increased
°	Degrees
📖	Book
AA	Alcoholics Anonymous
AADD	Adult Attention Deficit Disorder
ADHD	Attention Deficient Hyper activity Disorder
AIMS	Abnormal Involuntary Movement Scale
AO	Assertive Outreach
AOT	Assertive Outreach Team
ASW	Approved Social Worker
AUS	Aftercare Under Supervision
BA	Behavioural Activation
BAS	Barnes Akathisia Scale
BDI	Beck Depression Inventory
BMI	Body Mass Index
BNF	British National Formulary
BPRS	Brief Psychiatric Rating Scale
DBRS	Dangerous Behaviour Rating Scale
DBT	Dialectic Behaviour Therapy
DoH	Department of Health
DSM IV	Diagnostic and Statistical Manual
CAMI	Carers Assessment and Managing Index
CBT	Cognitive Behaviour Therapy
CCNAP	Community Care Needs Assessment Project
CMHN	Community Mental Health Nurse
CMHT	Community Mental Health Team
CMHTOP	Community Mental Health Team Older People
CMP	Clinical Management Plans
COP	Code of Practice
CPA	Care Programme Approach
CPN	Community Psychiatric Nurse
CSAP	Critical Skills Appraisal Programme

ECT	Electro Convulsive Therapy
ENDS	Evaluation of Nursing Documentation Schedule
ESC	Essential Shared Capabilities
FRASE	Falls Risk Assessment for the Elderly
GP	General Practitioner
GSH	Guided Self Help
HCR 20	Historical Clinical Risk Management (20 item scale)
HoNOS	Health of the Nation Outcome Scale
HR	Human Resources
HT	Humanistic Therapy
ICD	International Classification of Disease
IPT	Inter Personal Psychotherapy
IT	Information Technology
JCP	Joint Crisis Plans
KSF	Knowledge and Skills Framework
LMHN	Liaison Mental Health Nurse
MACA	Mental Aftercare Association (superseded by Together: working for wellbeing)
MAOI	Monoamine Uptake Inhibitors
MHA	Mental Health Act
MHAC	Mental Health Act Commission
MHRT	Mental Health Review Tribunal
MRSA	Methicillin Resistant Staphylococcus Aureus
NICE	National Institute for Clinical Excellence (superseded by NIHCE)
NIHCE	National Institute for Health and Clinical excellence
NHS	National Health Service
NMC	Nursing and Midwifery Council
NSF	National Service Framework
NSFMH	National Service Framework Mental Health
NSFOP	National Service Framework Older People
NOS	National Occupational Standards
OCD	Obsessive Compulsive Disorder
ODMP	Office of the Deputy Prime Minister
PALS	Patient Advice and Liaison Service
PCL	Psychopathy Check List
PD	Personality Disorder
PREP	Post Registration Education and Practice
PSI	Psycho Social Interventions
PTSD	Post Traumatic Stress Disorder
RCT	Randomised Control Trial

REM	Rapid Eye Movement
RMO	Registered Medical Officer
RO	Reality Orientation
RR	Rational Recovery
SAM	Suicide Assessment and Management
SAP	Single Assessment Process
SAS	Simpson Angus Scale
SCOFF	Sick, Control, One, Fat, Food
SEC	Side Effect Checklist
SFS	Social Functioning Scale
SHA	Strategic Health Authority
SMART	Specific, Measurable, Achievable, Realistic, Time orientated
SMI	Seriously Mentally Ill
SNRI	Selective Noradrenaline Reuptake Inhibitors
SOAS-R	Staff Observation of Aggression Scale
SP	Supportive Psychotherapy
SSRO	Selective Serotonin Reuptake Inhibitors
STRATIFY	St Thomas's Risk Assessment Tool in Falling Elderly Inpatients
TCA	Tricyclic Antidepressants
UK	United Kingdom
UKCC	United Kingdom Central Council (superseded by the NMC)
VRAG	Violence Risk Appraisal Guide
WHO	World Health Organization

Introduction

Concepts of mental health and illness

The most common and international definition of health was produced by the World Health Organization (WHO) in 1946. They defined 'health as a state of complete physical, mental and social well-being and not merely the absence of disease or infirmity'.[1] This definition of health relates not only to our minds and our bodies but also to our quality of life – including families, friends, and communities.

Although not without its critics, this definition can also be a starting point for thinking about the concept of mental health – it refers not only to our interior mental well-being but also to the quality of how we live our lives.

A concept can be defined as an abstract thought or idea. There is no one concept of mental health, but several categories of approach that have informed the thinking and delivery of mental health and illness care over the years.

The medical concept

The medical concept was developed by psychiatrists. They perceive the ill person as the problem, and believe that illness stems from a chemical imbalance within the brain. The focus for treatment has been on chemical intervention in the form of medication or psychosurgery. This concept is often criticized for ignoring social or familial links.

The anti-psychiatry concept

This concept stems from the work of T Szasz (1961).[2] He proposed that the experiences and behaviours referred to as mental illness were really problems associated with living, and an individual's inability to adapt to the world around them. Whilst Szasz acknowledged that some behaviour has a physical cause – such as acquired brain injury – he concludes that psychiatrists are oppressors and that there is no such thing as mental illness. He has been criticized for ignoring the genuine suffering of those with mental illness.

The family concept

R Laing (1964) contributed to this debate,[3] believing that the family was the cause of mental illness, particularly schizophrenia. He regarded the family as a pathogenic institution, unable to give a consistent approach to a child. Hence the child grows up unable to please the parents and suffering intolerable emotional stress, leading to mental illness. He proposed that psychiatrists colluded with the family in an attempt to control behaviour that others find a nuisance (Family therapy).

Helen Waldock, Health and Social Care Advisory Service

The labelling concept

Also in the 1960s, it was proposed by T Scheff[4] that labelling was the single most important cause of mental illness, in that you become what you are labelled. He was of the view that certain bizarre or 'deviant' behaviors which did not already fit into a defined category such as 'punk rocker' or 'Goth' (1960s examples being teddy boy or mod), were labelled mental illness. As a consequence, psychiatric symptoms can be seen as instances of residual deviancy which have become part of society's cultural stereotype of mental illness.

This concept helped by drawing attention to the notion of stigmatization of the mentally ill, although Scheff was criticized as the majority of people who become psychiatric patients suffer serious mental disturbances before any label is applied to them.

Psychoanalytical concepts

There are many and varied concepts in this category that understand us from the view of our unconscious and our early childhood experience. Freud's psychodynamic structure of personality suggests that behaviour is influenced by id, ego, and super ego, We are born id and our personality develops in stages during childhood. If there are conflicts associated with a particular phase of personality development (oral, anal, phallic latent, and genital) then fixations can develop that show themselves in personality. Jung and Ericson developed the broader psychodynamic approach believing that it is the social world that influences personality development.

Other concepts include attachment theory which explores the impact of early relationships with the primary carer (typically the mother). The bond between mother and child, or lack of bond, is thought to impact on the child's ability to engage with the world. At the heart of the theory lies a paradox in that children with very close attachments to the mother are also the most able to express their independence. Freudian concepts suggested that failure to break this attachment results in emotional trauma that could lead to later mental illness (☐ see Chapter 3 on Interventions).

References

1 World Health Organization. Constitution. WHO: Geneva, 1964.
2 Szasz, T. The Myth of Mental Illness. Harper: New York, 1961.
3 Laing, R, Easterton A. Sanity, Madness and the Family. Tavistock: London, 1964.
4 Scheff, T. Being Mentally Ill: A Sociological Theory. Aldine: Chicago, 1966.

Further reading (the classics)

Gabbard, G, Beck, JS, Holmes, J. Oxford Textbook of Psychotherapy. Oxford University Press: Oxford, 2005.
Holmes, J. John Bowlby and Attachment Theory. Routledge: London, 1993.
Pilgrim, D. Key Concepts in Mental Health. Sage Publications: Lodon, 2005.

Explaining mental illness

Recent years have seen many changes in the provision of services and therapies for people suffering from a range of mental health problems. The move away from large-scale institutional care to individual care in the community has been accompanied by a growth in the research and practice of evidence-based psychosocial approaches to care. The pharmaceutical industry has also contributed to current practice with the development of more refined user-friendly medications.

Although the exact cause of mental illness is not known, it is becoming clearer through research that many conditions are precipitated by a combination of biological, psychological, and environmental factors.

Biological Factors

- Abnormal balance of neurotransmitters: nerve cell chemicals enable brain cells to communicate with each other. When neurotransmitters are out of balance or not working properly, symptoms of mental illness can develop.
- Genetics: some mental illness runs in families and is passed on through genes. Rather than one gene causing a mental illness, it is thought that a person inherits susceptibility (multiple gene involvement), which when coupled with other factors, can trigger symptoms of mental illness.
- Infections: can be linked to brain damage and the development of mental illness, or the worsening of symptoms e.g. autoimmune neuro-psychiatric disorder has been linked to the development of OCD in children (📖 Obsessive compulsive disorder).
- Brain injury: cause may be prenatal, birth trauma, exposure to toxins, or acquired brain injury. All may contribute to the development of symptoms as the neurotransmitter pathways are disturbed.

Psychological factors

- Severe psychological trauma as a child e.g. emotional, physical, or sexual abuse.
- A significant early loss e.g. of a parent, sibling.
- Emotional or physical neglect.
- Poor ability to relate to others.

Environmental factors

- A dysfunctional family life.
- Death or divorce.
- Poverty.
- Feelings of inadequacy, low self esteem, anxiety, anger, or loneliness.
- Changing jobs or school.
- Social or cultural expectations.
- Substance misuse by an individual or their parents.

Helen Waldock, Health and Social Care Advisory Service

Although all individuals react in different ways to different events, there are some groups in society that are exposed to more stressors than others. These include migrants, refugees, and asylum seekers, those who live in extreme poverty, and those who have no true sense of self. These people are more vulnerable to developing mental illness, hence the reason for accurate and corroborated history taking.

Further reading

Kuipers, E, Bebbington, P. *Living with Mental Illness: a book for relatives and friends*. Souvenir Press: UK, 2005.

Further viewing (available on DVD)

A Beautiful Mind, Directed by Ron Howard, produced by Brain Grazer and Ron Howard. Distributed by Universal Pictures. Length 134 minutes.
The Snake Pit, Directed by Anatole Litvak, produced by Robert Bassler, Anatole Litvak & Darryl Zanuck. Distributed by 20th Century Fox. Length 108 minutes.

Understanding mental illness

Mental illness refers collectively to all diagnosable mental disorders characterized by alterations in thinking, mood, or behaviour or a combination of these, mediated by the brain and associated with distress and impaired functioning. There have been concerted efforts to develop systems for classifying mental illness that would be relevant for use across cultures. Two classification systems are used:

1) Diagnostic and Statistical Manual of Mental Illness (DSM IV)[5]
2) Diagnostic and Statistical Manual of Mental and Behavioural disorders referred to as ICD 10 (International Classification of Disease version 10)—this is the classification system used primarily in the UK.[6]

Both the above have gone some way to providing uniformity and consistency to the diagnosis and classification of mental illness, however they are not without their critics.

Parker *et al.* (1995) said they 'failed to represent the diversity of the human experiences of distress'.[7] He also argues that these systems fail to take account of race, identity, gender, and social power. They are in themselves social constructs developed by the western world, and based on the medical model.

These classification systems do have their place as they help to determine the severely ill from the moderate or mildly ill. The absence of such systems would hamper the ability to plan services, evaluate treatments or interventions, or evaluate the effectiveness of preventative strategies.[8]

We may all suffer from one or more of the symptoms described in either classification system at some point in our life. It is unhelpful, meaningless, and stigmatizing to have personal distress labelled in such a manner that people respond to the label rather that the individual. This can be demonstrated by the comparison in the table opposite.

It is more important to understand the experience of the person living with mental ill-health rather than attempting to understand mental illness *per se.*

Note:

Co-morbidity – refers to the existence of two or more illnesses in the same individual.

Serious Mental Illness (SMI) refers to people who have an illness that is long lasting and severely interferes with a person's ability to participate in life activities.

Helen Waldock, Health and Social Care Advisory Service

Comparison of the psychosocial and biomedical perspectives

Criteria	Psychosocial	Biomedical
Cause of illness	Behaviour, beliefs, poverty, coping mechanisms, relationships, childhood trauma	Genetics, brain injury, viral or bacterial infection, birth trauma, neurotransmitter imbalance
Responsibility for illness	Individual, social, political, environmental factors, economics	External forces causing internal change
Treatment of illness	Holistic approach: change in beliefs, coping style, economic status, relationships	Medication or other medical intervention, surgery, ECT (📖 ECT)
Responsibility for treatment	Individual, family, significant other, support networks	The doctor and other professional involved in collaboration with the individual
Relationship between mental health and illness	Both exist on a continuum, with degrees of mental health and mental illness	Dichotomous, the person is either healthy or ill
Relationship between mind and body	The mind and body are mutually interdependent	The mind and body function independently of one another
Role in health and illness	Psychosocial factors contribute to an individual's mental health status	Illness has psychosocial consequences not causes

References

5 American Psychiatric Association. Diagnostic and Statistical Manual of Mental Disorders, 4th revision. American Psychiatric Press U.S.A 1994.

6 World Health Organization. International Classification of Mental and Behavioural Disorders, 10th revision. WHO: Geneva, 1992.

7 Parker, I, Geogarca E, Harper D, McLaughlin T and Stowell-Smith M. Deconstructing Psychopathology. Sage: London, 1995.

8 Newton, J. Preventing Mental Illness. Routledge: London, 1988.

The stress vulnerability model

The stress vulnerability model is of considerable importance in mental Health Nursing (MHN). It was first described in an article written nearly 30 years ago.[9] This article suggested that a vulnerability to schizophrenia was made up of:

- Variables which could be described as 'inborn', such as genes.
- Variables which could be described as 'acquired', which may include physical events (e.g. perinatal complications and illnesses such as influenza during pregnancy), developmental phenomena, and various life events.

This model has been developed and adapted over the years, and has received some criticism. However, it is of considerable practical use because it embraces a wide range of research demonstrating a wide spectrum of causative factors. It overcomes rather sterile debates about the causation and maintenance of mental illnesses, particularly schizophrenia and other psychoses.

How can the mental health nurse use this model?

This model is particularly useful for the mental health nurse when dealing with people with existing illnesses – particularly schizophrenia and other psychoses – as it recognizes that stress may lead to relapse. The mental health nurse may be very effective in preventing relapse by:

- Helping the person deal with stresses from a range of sources e.g. by anxiety management training, or by teaching the person to cope with hallucinations.
- Providing interventions which deal with the stress itself e.g. family interventions in schizophrenia or interventions for substance abuse.

Relapse is often triggered by a combination of stresses such as boredom, drug use, the stigma attached to the illness and a negative family environment, rather than a single stress.[10] The mental health nurse is ideally placed to deliver a wide range of interventions which can be described as 'psychosocial'; and training in these interventions is now offered to most of these nurses who work in the community (📖 Psychosocial interventions).

Although this model is clearly applicable to the practical management of most mental health problems, as noted above, it has been largely applied to schizophrenia. Research now clearly demonstrates that there is an inborn or acquired vulnerability to a range of conditions, including depression, anxiety, and obsessive compulsive disorder. Other disorders may be triggered by the influence of various stressors.

Professor Kevin Gournay Institute of Psychiatry, Kings College, London

References

 9 Zubin, J, Spring, B. Vulnerability: A new view of schizophrenia. *Journal of Abnormal Psychology*
86: 260–6, 1977.
10 Warner, R. *Recovery from schizophrenia*, 2nd edn. Routledge: London, 1994.

The experience of mental illness

Mental illness is associated with a significant burden of morbidity and disability. Lifetime rates for any kind of psychological disorder are higher, affecting nearly half the population.[11] Mental disorders are often undiagnosed by doctors, and people are reluctant to seek professional help.

Overall rates of psychiatric disorders are the same for men as they are for women but there are distinctions in the patterns:

- Unipolar depression is twice as common in women (📖 Depression).
- Men are three times more likely to be diagnosed with an antisocial personality disorder (📖 Personality disorder).
- There are no marked differences in severe mental illnesses between men and women.
- Less than 2% of the population have a severe mental illness 📖 Schizophrenia.

The experience of mental illness is unique to each individual regardless of the symptoms they are suffering, due to the individual experience of emotion. For example the vast majority of people have felt 'happiness' at some point in their lives, some cried at this time and others laughed.

Common symptoms experienced

Mood changes

- **Anxiety:** this is greater than the tension felt in a stressful situation, such as exams. It is characterized by physical symptoms such as palpitations, sweating, tremor, and the fear that something awful is about to happen (📖 Anxiety).
- **Depression:** this is greater than the accepted response to a sad or tragic life event. It is typical to have disturbed sleep, reduced appetite, little interest in life, feeling hopeless and helpless.
- **Elation:** this is greater than excitement, and is coupled with irritability and impatience. A person's view of themselves may also be altered e.g. by becoming grand and extravagant both materially and personally.

📖 Bipolar disorder

Thought processes

- Delusions; these are greater than just being wrong. It is a belief or impression that is absolute and unshakable, not open to change through experience or discussion. Examples are persecutory delusions, where a person feels they are being 'got at', or delusions of reference, where a person believes that the TV, radio, or newspapers are referring specifically to them.
- Obsessional or compulsive thoughts: these are greater than everyday routines that we all have, or set ways of doing certain tasks. These thoughts are intrusive, unwanted, and beyond a person's control. They may be coupled with repetitive behaviour (ritualistic behaviour) that cannot be interrupted.

Helen Waldock, Health and Social Care Advisory Service

- Odd thoughts: these are greater than the occasional sense of deja-vu experienced by many. It is when a person thinks that others can read/see into their mind (thought broadcast) or are able to put their thoughts into the mind of others (thought insertion).
📖 Schizophrenia

Perceptual changes

This refers to how an individual experiences the world around them and their unique sense of reality. In mental illness, there are sometimes changes to these experiences that are very real to the individual, but not experienced by anyone else. These experiences are referred to as hallucinations:

- *Auditory:* where voice/voices/conversations/noise that do not belong to the individual are heard within a person's head (most common).
- *Visual:* where a person sees things that are not seen by anyone else.
- *Olfactory:* where a person can smell something that is not smelt by anyone else.
- *Tactile:* where a person can feel something, usually on their skin, that is not connected to any external stimuli.
- *Gustatory:* where a person experiences a particular taste that is not related to anything in their surroundings.

Behaviour changes

These may be marked and varied depending on other symptoms experienced by the person. They sometimes result in poor self-care to the extent of neglect. They are not symptoms in themselves but an indicator that all may not be well.

Speech changes

If thoughts, perception, and mood changes are occurring, then it is logical that a person's speech will change, not only in what they say but in how they say it. They may lose or have exaggerated intonation, or they may struggle to communicate at all. They may keep changing the subject (flight of ideas), or speak so quickly that they are difficult to follow or stop (pressure of speech).

Reference

11 World Health Organization. *The world health statistics annual.* WHO: Geneva, 1995.

Further Reading

Jampolsky, L. *Walking Through the Walls.* Celestial Arts Berkeley, California 2005.

Tessler, RC, Gamache, C. *Family Experiences with Mental Illness.* Auburn House Publishing Company, Westport, CT 2000.

Wahl OF. *Telling is a Risky Business: the experience of mental illness and stigma.* Rutgers University Press: Piscataway NJ, 2000.

Early detection of mental illness

For people of all ages, early detection, assessment, and linkage with treatment and supports can prevent mental health problems from resulting in poor life outcomes. Different behaviours are characteristic for different stages of life. The focus of early detection is on patterns of behaviour. Physical health problems need to be excluded before considering mental illness.

In children and adolescents the onset of illness is usually gradual and it is often difficult to establish if they are going through a temporary phase. The following signs can indicate many things, but if they persist, they may indicate the onset of a mental illness and a thorough assessment by a mental health professional is recommended.

Changes in younger children
- Clear change in school performance.
- Misuse of alcohol and/or drugs.
- Inability to cope with problems and daily activities.
- Marked changes in sleeping and/or eating habits.
- Many complaints of physical ailments e.g. headaches.
- Aggressive or non-aggressive consistent infringement of rights of others.
- Opposition to authority including truancy, thefts, or vandalism.
- Strong fear of becoming obese with no relationship to actual body weight.
- Depression shown by continued, protracted negative mood and attitude, often accompanied by poor appetite, difficulty sleeping, or thoughts of death.
- Recurrent outbursts of anger. Self-injurious behavior e.g. head-banging, self-biting, cutting.

Changes in pre-adolescents and adolescents
- Clear change in school performance.
- Misuse of alcohol and/or drugs.
- Inability to cope with problems and daily activities.
- Marked changes in sleeping and/or eating habits.
- Many complaints of physical ailments e.g. headaches.
- Aggressive or non-aggressive consistent infringement of rights of others.
- Opposition to authority including truancy, thefts, or vandalism.
- Strong fear of becoming obese with no relationship to actual body weight.
- Depression shown by continued, protracted negative mood and attitude, often accompanied by poor appetite, difficulty sleeping, or thoughts of death.
- Recurrent outbursts of anger.
- Self-injurious behavior e.g. head-banging, self-biting, cutting.

Helen Waldock, Health and Social Care Advisory Service

Changes in adults

- Withdrawal and loss of interest in usual activities.
- Loss of energy or motivation.
- Problems with memory and concentration.
- Deterioration in work or study.
- Lack of emotional response or inappropriate emotional display.
- Sleep or appetite disturbances.
- Unusual ideas or behaviours.
- Feeling 'changed' in some way.

Changes in the older person (early dementia)

- Recent memory loss that affects employment and social activity
  e.g. names and people.
- Difficulty performing familiar tasks e.g. cooking, cleaning.
- Problems with language e.g. forgetting simple words.
- Disorientation to time and familiar places e.g. own street.
- Poor or decreased judgments e.g. driving ability.
- Problems with abstract thinking e.g. not recognizing symbols such as £.
- Misplacing things e.g. putting door keys in the fridge.
- Changes in mood or behaviour unrelated to events.
- Changes in personality e.g. stops communicating.
- Loss of initiative e.g. does not get dressed.

Further reading

Cooper, M. Child and Adolescent Mental Health. Hodder Education: 2005. UK
Salovey, PR and Rothman AJ. The Social Psychology of Health. Taylor Francis Ltd. UK. 2003.

The Capable Practitioner Framework (CPF)

Mental health practitioners are facing the greatest and fastest moving set of changes encountered for several decades, courtesy of the National Service Frameworks (NSF).[12] (📖 National Service Frameworks)

The changing arena of service provision is now more varied, dispersed, and complex than ever before. The requirements for effective care now come from numerous agencies such as primary care, housing, social services, the voluntary sector, and the family, as well as specialist mental health services, creating problems of coordination, accountability, and efficiency. Service provision has been re-orientated to put the requirements of the service user/family/carer at its centre, and the increasing development of evidence-based interventions has created the need for the capable practitioner.

The capable practitioner is a broad, unifying, theoretical framework which encompasses the set of skills, knowledge, and attitudes required within the work force of mental health practitioners to effectively implement the national service framework. They are not the domain of any one of the professions and are developed as part of pre- and post-registration/qualifying training.

Capability can be defined as:
- A performance component: identifying what people need to possess in the way of knowledge, skills, and attitude, and what they need to achieve in the work place.
- An ethical component: integrating knowledge of culture, values, and social awareness into professional practice.
- An emphasis on reflective practice in action.
- The ability to effectively implement evidence-based interventions in the modern mental health system.
- A commitment to working with new models of professional practice and responsibility for life-long learning.

The capability framework combines the notions of a reflective practitioner with that of an effective practitioner. The process moves from a base where all the workforce must have ethical practice moving through the five domains to increasing specialism that will only apply to some staff.

Five domains for modern mental health practice:
1. Ethical Practice: makes assumptions about the values and attitudes needed for practice.
2. Knowledge: recognized as being the foundation of effective practice.
3. Process of care: describes the capabilities required to work effectively in partnership with users, carers, families, team members, and other agencies.
4. Interventions: these are capabilities specific to a particular evidence base within mental health care.
5. Context specific application e.g. assertive outreach, home treatment, crisis resolution.
📖 Shared capabilities

Helen Waldock, Health and Social Care Advisory Service

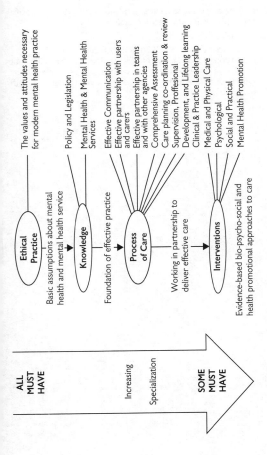

Fig.1.1 A framework for capable practice (SCMM 2001).

Each of these five categories is further subdivided to arrive at specific statements of capability for mental health practice.

Other competency frameworks

Knowledge and skills framework (KSF): NHS-only focus.[13]

National Occupational Standards (NOS): similar to the CPF but designed to provide a measurement of output or performance by detailed descriptions of competence required in providing mental health services.[14]

📖 NOS

References

12 National Service Framework Mental Health 1999 Department of Health. The Stationary Office London.
13 Department of Health. Knowledge and Skills Framework. DoH: London, 2004. www.dh.gov.uk
14 National Institute for Mental Health England. National Occupational Standards. NIMHE: London, 2003. www.nihme.org.uk.

Further reading

Sainsbury's Centre for Mental Health. The Capable Practitioner. SCMH London 2001. www.scmh.org.uk.

Person-centred mental health nursing

The National Service Framework for Mental Health (1999) set out the principles for contemporary mental health care in England. Central to this is the Care Programme Approach (CPA) (📖 CPA). For the CPA to be effective the service user must be well informed about mental health and mental health services, they must be at the centre of their own care, in partnership with staff and able to exercise informed choice.

The principles of person-centred care are:

The service user

- Should be informed about services and how to access them, in clear language of their choice (including sign language) (📖 Enabling access to mental health services).
- Will have their views and wishes at the forefront throughout assessment, care planning, and service delivery.
- Be given an assessment that not only identifies what is needed, but takes account of their strengths and abilities (📖 Mental Health assessment).
- Expects processes and services to enable maximum potential for independence (📖 Rehabilitation and recovery).
- Must be involved in decisions about their care and be empowered to determine the level of risk they are prepared to take.
- Be given realistic options as to how their needs can be met within existing eligibility criteria.
- Consent to information being collected about them and agreeing how this may be shared.
- When somebody lacks the capacity to make decisions to give consent, services must secure their maximum participation whilst safe-guarding their interests.
- Should receive high quality care that is evidence based, efficient, non-discriminatory, tailored to their individual needs, and acceptable to them.

The carers and the family

- Can be involved with the care of the individual if they chose to be, and where the individual has given consent.
- Have their support needs as a carer assessed in their own right.
- Be supported and educated in the care they give.
- Treated with the same respect, consideration and non-discrimination as the service user.

📖 Providing mental health services which support families and carers

Integrated services (📖 CPA)

- Access to services is via a coordinated and straightforward assessment, with duplication kept to a minimum.
- Effective information sharing, where confidentiality is respected, is crucial for effective person-centred care.

Helen Waldock, Health and Social Care Advisory Service

- Agencies must coordinate services in the best interests of the individual.
- Promoting health and well-being is an integral part of the service to the individual.
- Rehabilitation and recovery should be the models of choice.

Staff

- Should receive proper training and development to adapt to the changing mental health climate.
- Have the right to clinical and professional supervision (📖 Clinical supervision).
- Receive an annual appraisal and continuing professional development – these are integral to valuing staff (📖 Management supervision).

Further reading

Adams, N. *Treatment Planning for Person-Centred Care: the road to mental health and addiction recovery.* Academic Press: London 2004.

Benson WD, Briscoe L. Jumping the Hurdles of Mental Health Care Wearing Cement Shoes. *Journal of American Psychiatric Nurses Association* **9**: 123–8, 2003.

Bryant-Jeffe, R. *Responding to a Serious Mental Health Problem: person-centred dialogues.* Radcliffe Medical Press: 2005.

The principles and codes of professional practice

All professions provide their own code for professional practice whether they are delivering clinical care or managing services. The purpose of a code of practice is to enable clarity on the basic standards that service users can expect. They ensure that services are provided in a legal and ethical manner by adhering to established protocols, procedures, and guidelines. All codes of practice contain the same fundamental underlying principles:

- To place the needs of service users ahead of the professionals own agenda.
- To promote health and prevent illness.
- To maintain confidentiality in keeping with the law.
- To respect the right to life or death with dignity.
- To respect individuality, regardless of age, race, disability, culture, gender orientation, politics, nationality, or social status.
- To reduce or alleviate suffering with empathy.
- To take personal responsibility and accountability for your practice.
- To act in a manner that promotes the profession.
- To cooperate with other professionals in the delivery of care.

Further detail can be explored by subdividing into key relationships between the profession, the service user, practice, the profession, and colleagues (see table opposite).

Inherent within these principles is the notion of 'Duty of care'.

Duty of care requires that everything possible is done to protect the health and safety of others, whether they are service users or staff.

Individual professions can access their code of practice from the home page of their professional body. For registered nurses in the UK: www.nmc-uk.org.uk.

Key concepts of professional practice include:

Compassion: the humane quality of understanding the suffering of others and wanting to do something about it.

Integrity: the characteristics of honesty and sincerity.

Empowerment: the process of increasing personal, interpersonal, and political power to enable individuals or collectives to improve their life situation. It requires the full participation of people in the formulation, implementation and evaluation of decisions determining the functioning and well-being of society.

Helen Waldock, Health and Social Care Advisory Service

Roles & Responsibilites

Practitioners and service users	Practitioners and practice	Practitioners and the profession	Practitioners and colleagues
Provide care that respects human rights and is individual	Set standards of care which promote best practice and quality	Set standards for practice, education, research, and management	Support workplace systems to promote MD working
Provide adequate information to promote informed choice and consent	Take responsibility for maintaining registration or licence	Support the dissemination of research- and practice-based evidence	Ensure that people and the environment are fit for the purpose
Treat service users with integrity and competence	Strive to improve professional skills of self and other team members	Advance and protect the standards of the profession	Support a culture that promotes common ethical values
Ensure clinical and environmental safety	Promote the utilization of evidence-based practice	Evaluate the quality of work against professional standards	Safeguard individuals and the community from poor practice

Further reading

Blais K, Mayes J, Kozier B. *Professional Nursing Practice, Concepts and Perspectives*. Prentice-Hall: New Jersy 2005.
Davies, C, Filay, JL. *Changing Practice in Health and Social Care*, Sage Publications: London, 2000.

Accountability

Originally accountability referred to the compliance with the established norms of financial management. More recently, the meaning of accountability has broadened to include the achievement of performance targets, such as those outlined in the National Service Frameworks, and with norms external to the organisation, such as the Human Rights Act 📖 NSF.

Within health care environments there are three clear levels of accountability:

Personal accountability

At its most general, accountability is about an individual who is responsible for a set of activities explaining or answering for their actions. In a hierarchical environment such as the Health Service, it is associated with delegated authority, and is distinct from responsibility. For example, the Chief Executive is ultimately accountable for the organization, but is not responsible for individual actions of staff or service users (called vicarious liability).

Professional accountability

Here there are two strands to accountability, firstly to the service user, and secondly to colleagues. Traditionally, accountability has focused on competence, and on legal and ethical conduct as determined by professional bodies, such as the Nursing and Midwifery Council or the General Medical Council. These bodies establish the content areas that determine competence, but it is not possible for them to monitor an individual's practice. Colleagues are therefore accountable for enforcing professional standards of practice. More recently, accountability to individual service users has become more prominent.
📖 Principles and codes of professional practice.

Organizational accountability

This comprises the entire management and control of an organization, including its organizational structure, its business policy, its principles, and guidelines, with both internal and external monitoring being mandatory. It is sometimes referred to as corporate governance or corporate accountability for clinical practice. Within health care, **Clinical Governance** is the major framework through which the organization is held accountable to the public and to the government. This is a systematic approach to maintaining and improving the quality of patient care. It is a multi-disciplinary, multi-agency activity that covers seven domains. These domains are not held in isolation but are networked throughout the organizations to produce a seamless service.

Helen Waldock, Health and Social Care Advisory Service

Domains of clinical governance (📖 Clinical governance).

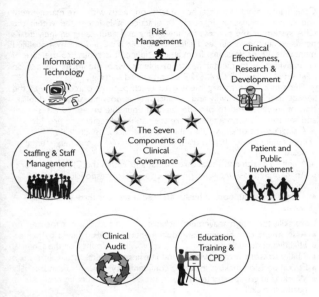

Fig.1.2 Domains of clinical governance www.chi.nhs.uk.

Further reading

McSherry, R, Graham-Brown, R. *Clinical Governance: a guide to implementation for Healthcare Professionals.* Blackwell Publishing: Oxford, 2002.

Tiley, S, Watson, R. *Accountability in Nursing and Midwifery*, Blackwell Publishing: Oxford, 2003.

Case management skills

Case management in mental health is synonymous with care management and care coordination. In terms of practice, it is integrated within the CPA system as the process for identifying and addressing an individual's needs within the resources available. The role is carried out by a qualified mental health professional from any discipline. It is central to the care of an individual with mental health problems, with the focus on person centred planning (📖 CPA, 📖 Person-centred nursing).

The aim of case management is to reach positive outcomes with the service user as effectively and as efficiently as possible, to avoid duplication of services, and to provide fair and equitable access to assessment and services. To support this, there are national directives to provide:

• A single point of entry to mental health services, usually via a community mental health team (📖 The effective community mental health team).
• A unified health and social care assessment within the CPA framework.
• An identified case manager or care coordinator responsible for all agencies involved.
• Access to the support of health and social services through a single point.

Core skills for case management include:
• Assessment, care planning, and documentation skills.
• Effective communication.
• Ability to work with individuals and families or carers.
• Ethical decision-making, including confidentiality.
• Working in groups and teams.
• Leadership skills.
• Intervention skills: influencing, interviewing, enabling, involving.
• Navigational skills: systems, procedures, protocols, eligibility criteria.
• Creative and lateral thinking.
• Analytical skills.
• Emotional intelligence.

Helen Waldock, Health and Social Care Advisory Service

The core role of a case manager

Three whats?	Three hows?
COLLECT data from service user, family, and others involved	COP – define and negotiate the non-negotiable
CREATE a care plan with the service user	COACH – teach new skills to service user and other agencies
COORDINATE with care partners to ensure delivery of the care plan	CONSULTANT– provide information for education and to enable others to make informed decisions

Efficacy of case management

There is little formal research into the efficacy of case management although emerging results indicate:
- Increased numbers remaining in contact with services.
- Increased numbers admitted to psychiatric hospital.
- Possible increases the length of stay in hospital.
- Some improvement in compliance, medication, and activities.
- No significant improvement of mental state, social functioning, or quality of life.
- Potentially more expensive than traditional case work.

📖 Following through on care programmes for people with mental health needs.

Further reading

Building Bridges – a guide to arrangements for inter-agency working for the protection of severely mentally ill people. HSG(95)96 Department of Health 1995. The Stationery Office London.

Care management and assessment – Practioners Guide. Department of Health 1991 The Stationery Office London.

Effective Care Coordination in Mental Health – Modernising the CPA. Department of Health. The Stationery Office London 1999.

Values and attitudes for professional practice

A value is a belief or an ideal to which an individual is committed. It is an important part of the base or foundation of a profession, and is often connected to the reasoning behind practice, procedure, and policy. Attitudes reflect the values of an individual or an organization, and can be a positive or negative response to an object, person, concept, or a situation.

Vales and attitudes can be organized around seven key concepts and can form the basis for a profession's philosophy:

- *Altruism* – unselfish concern for the welfare of others.
- *Dignity* – valuing the inherent worth and uniqueness of an individual.
- *Equality* – individuals are perceived as having fundamental human rights and opportunities, and should be treated with fairness and impartiality.
- *Truth* – requires adherence to accurate facts when working with service users, colleagues, and the public.
- *Justice* -placing value on the upholding of moral and legal principles such as fairness, equality, truthfulness, and objectivity.
- *Freedom* – refers to the exercise of informed choice, independence, and self direction.
- *Prudence* – the ability to govern and discipline oneself.

Attitudes and values are learnt as an individual travels through life, from friends, family, leaders, influential people, experience, culture, race, and religion. The formation of professional values and beliefs is an important part of professional socialization, and will impact on professional practice. The 'Six Pillars of Character'[15] developed by the Josephson Institute of Ethics, identifies the constructs for professional behaviour and practice:

Reference

15 Josephson Institute of Ethics. Six Pillars of Character. Josephson Institute of Ethics: www.josephsoninstitute.org California.

Further reading

Green, C. Critical Thinking in Nursing: case studies across the curriculum. Prentice Hall: New Jersey, 2000.

Katz, JR, Carter C, Bishop J, Kravits S. Keys to Nursing Success. Prentice Hall: New Jersey. 2003.

Helen Waldock, Health and Social Care Advisory Service

Character Attributes (values and attitude)	Description (behaviour)
Trustworthiness	Do what you say you are going to do
	A person who is trustworthy exhibits the following behaviours:
	Acts with integrity
	Is honest and does not deceive
	Keeps a promise
	Is consistent
	Is loyal to those who are not present
	Is reliable
	Is credible
	Has a good reputation
Respect	Treat others the way they treat you
	A person who is respectful exhibits the following behaviours:
	Is open and tolerant of differences
	Is considerate and courteous
	Deals peacefully with anger/disagreements/insults
	Treats others the way they want to be treated
Responsibility	Do what you are supposed to do
	A person who is responsible exhibits the following behaviours:
	Acts with self discipline
	Thinks before they act
	Understands that actions create consequences
	Is consistent
	Is accountable
Fairness	Play by the rules
	A person who is fair exhibits the following behaviours:
	Is open minded
	Listens to others
	Shares information
	Does not needlessly blame others
	Is equitable and impartial
Caring	Show you care
	A person who cares exhibits the following behaviours:
	Expresses gratitude to others
	Forgives others
	Helps people in need
	Is compassionate
Citizenship	Do your share
	A person who is a good citizen exhibits the following behaviours:
	Cooperates
	Stays informed
	Is a good neighbour
	Protects the environment
	Obeys the law
	Exhibits civil duty
	Seeks the common good for most people

The carer's charter

In this context 'carer' does not mean care worker or care staff who are paid to provide care as part of employment, rather those people who look after a relative or friend when they are unwell or distressed. At some point in our life we will all require care of one sort or another, and we will probably all give care at some point.

According to the 2001 census, 5.2 million people were providing unpaid informal care in England and Wales. This number does not take into account young carers or parent carers. Caring is often not the only role these people have; 31% are in full-time employment.

The National Service Framework (NSF) for Mental Health, Standard 6, states that all carers who provide regular and substantial care for a person should:

- Have an assessment of their caring, physical, and mental health needs repeated on at least an annual basis.
- Have their own written care plan which is given to them and implemented in discussion with them.

📖 Providing mental health Services which support families and carers

What carers want

- Well-being for the person being cared for.
- Freedom to pursue their own interests.
- To remain fit and healthy.
- Involvement with, and confidence in the statutory and voluntary services.
- Choice in terms of formal care and support.
- Information to make informed choices and decisions.

Note: the extent of a carer's involvement depends on the consent of the service user, which can raise issues around confidentiality and conflict.

'Caring for Carers' is the National Strategy for England and Wales which has led to the development of local strategies and carer's charters outlining carer's rights, and is based on the following principles:

- Recognition of the carer's role and expertise.
- Giving the advice and information carers need to provide care.
- Recognizing, responding to and incorporating individual needs into the service users care plan.
- Offering help and support when needed.
- Being involved in the planning, development, and evaluation of services.

Local carers charters will represent the priorities of the carers in their area and may include specifics such as the Mental Health Act or advocacy.

On the Mental Health Act for example:

- Making information on the Mental Health Act freely available, both verbal and written.
- Giving information on your rights under the Mental Health Act.
- Being cared for with respect to the Human Rights Act.

📖 Mental Health Act

Helen Waldock, Health and Social Care Advisory Service

On advocacy, for example
• Including advocates in your care as you choose.
• Being given information or an explanation of the different forms of advocacy.
• Being informed of any available advocacy schemes and how to access them.
📖 Working with advocacy services

Further reading

Caring about carers a national strategy for carers. 1999. Department of Health, London. www.carers.gov.uk

Department of Health. Carers and Disabled Children's Act. DoH: London, 2000. www.dh.gov.uk

National Institute for Mental Health England. Valuing Carers – The Mental Health Carers Charter; A Guide for Carers; Working with Carers. NIMHE: London.

All at: www.nimhe.org

Guidelines for working with users

The government's NHS Plan[16] states that the Health Service should be more patient centred. The NHS and Social Care Act[17] demands that every NHS body has a statutory duty to consult and involve patients and the public in its activities.

In every NHS Trust there is a Patient's Advice and Liaison Service (PALS), to provide help and support for people about the Trusts services. This includes complaints procedures and advice about local voluntary and self-help groups. Independent and statutory forums or groups for patients or service users have been set up, to monitor and review services, as well as to influenece the day-to-day management of each Trust.

The Commission for Patient and Public Involvement (PPI) is an independent organization that collects, compares, and promotes information picked up through local networks, PALS, and Patient Forums. They have set national standards for the involvement of patients, and provide training to ensure that local volunteers and representatives are able to meet these standards. See www.cppih.org.uk

Principles for good practice:

- Be clear about what is wanted from service user and carers, as well as being clear about the role and responsibilities of others, professionals, carers, voluntary organizations, and so on.
- Be respectful of each other, as all have the right to express their own view.
- Be inclusive, by involving a diverse group that reflects the local population.
- Be flexible by adapting work practices, and accept that from time to time people's health may affect their ability to work.
- Be accessible by avoiding the use of jargon and using plain English.
- Offer resources and practical and emotional support to enable people to fulfil their role.
- Avoid tokenism, and enable people to give support and encouragement to others.
- Involve people at all stages of service delivery, development, and evaluation.

By working with service users, NHS Trusts can:

- Help ensure that services are more effective and efficient.
- Inform commissioners about gaps in services.
- Provide feedback on how service users experience local services.
- Provide a better picture of service users experiences, perceptions, and priorities.
- Ensure users get appropriate responses which meet their needs, and not the needs of the organization.
- Encourage the commissioning and development of a range of service provision options and choices.

Helen Waldock, Health and Social Care Advisory Service

Key areas for working with service user are:
- Involvement in service delivery and care including prioritization in care planning, where users actively participate in their Care Programme Approach (CPA) assessment.
- Involvement in strategic planning, e.g. involving both individuals and groups in activities for local improvement plans.
- Support and training for service users e.g. enabling the acquisition of skills and knowledge to support full participation on an equal footing in relation to mental health services and policy.
- Developing user-led and managed projects and forums, e.g. establishing user forums at a team level, or within a ward or community setting.
- Welcoming user feedback, e.g. involvement in the monitoring and evaluation of local services through the governance systems.
- Involving service users in the training, employment, and evaluation of staff.

References

16 Department of Health. The NHS Plan. DoH: London, 2000.
17 Department of Health. NHS and Social Care Bill. DoH: London, 1990.

Further reading

Tait L, Lester HE. Encouraging user involvement in mental health services. *Advances in Psychiatric Treatment* **11**: 168–75, 2005.

Ethics

Ethics is the general term for what is described as the science of morality. Philosophically, ethical behaviour is that which is right or good. In this instance, it is behaviour that conforms to professional practice. Ethics refers to principles that define behaviour as right, good and proper. Such principles do not always indicate a single 'moral' course of action, but provide a means of evaluating and deciding among competing options.

Ethical behaviour forms the basis of mental health care (📖 The capable practitioner). There are two main sources of ethical policy guidance for mental health practitioners:

1. The Code of Professional Conduct for Nurses and Midwives from the Nursing and Midwifery Council (NMC), is specifically for nurses.[18]
   The NMC have also produced specific guidelines for mental health. These are:
   - Guidelines for the administration of medication (2002).
   - Guidelines on practitioner-patient relationships and the prevention of abuse (2002).
   📖 Code of professional conduct

2. The Code of Practice to the Mental Health Act (1983). This was designed specifically to enable those with the authority to detain people under the Act, to behave in a morally and ethically responsible manner.
   📖 Mental Health Act

There are seven core values shared by all health care regulatory bodies that govern the ethical behaviour of practitioners:

- Respect the patient, the client, or service user as an individual.
- Obtain consent before giving any treatment or care (consent is an ongoing consideration and should be sought before every intervention).
- Protect confidential information.
- Cooperate with others in teams.
- Maintain professional knowledge and competence.
- Be trustworthy.
- Act to identify and minimise risk to patients, clients, or users.

Ethics is about putting principles into actions. Consistency between what we say we value, and what our actions say we value, is a matter of personal integrity (📖 Ethical issues in research).

Helen Waldock, Health and Social Care Advisory Service

The process of ethical decision-making requires:

Commitment	Consciousness	Competency
The desire to do the right thing regardless of cost to self – emotional, material, or physical	The awareness to act consistently and apply moral convictions to daily behaviour, in keeping with professional principles	The ability to collect and evaluate information, to develop alternatives, to see potential consequences and risks

Making ethical decisions: things to ask yourself:
• Does your decision conflict with any core ethical values?
• Think of someone whose moral judgement you respect. Would they make the same decision?
• How will your decision affect others?
• Are your actions legal? Have you checked?
• Are there regulations, rules, policies, or procedures that restrict your choices or actions? Have you read them?
• Would your decision be perceived as unethical?
• How would your decision look if it were reported in the media?
• Would you be proud of your decision if your child, sibling, or parent found out? Would you want them to make the same decision?
• Could you honestly defend your decision?
• Will you sleep soundly tonight?

Reference
18 Nursing and Midwifery Council. Code of Professional Conduct. NMC London: 2002. See also www.nmc.org for other guidelines.

Further reading
Department of Health. Good Practice in Consent. DoH: London, 2001 (HSC2001/023).
Jones, RM. Mental Health Act Manual, 8th edn. Swet & Maxwell: London, 2003.

The essence of care

The essence of care is about improving the aspects of care that are most important to service users. It is a patient-focused benchmarking toolkit that was first launched by the Chief Nursing Officer for England and Wales in 2001. Following its implementation across several pilot sites, the tool-kit was simplified, reviewed, and relaunched in 2003. It supports the Clinical Governance Framework.

As the essence of care is contained in the portfolio of the chief Nursing Officer, it is often viewed as being wholly within the domain of Nursing. This is not the reality, as the benchmarks or standards are applicable to all employees and all departments, not just the professions working within health and social services.

The essence of care is a continuous quality improvement cycle, using statements of best practice, and it is focused on patients or service users. The areas of care where standards have been set and benchmarking applies are:

- Continence, bladder, and bowel care
- Personal and oral hygiene
- Food and nutrition
- Pressure ulcers
- Privacy and dignity
- Record keeping
- Safety of all service users with mental health needs in acute mental health and general hospital settings
- Principles of self-care
- Communication.

These are not stand-alone areas and are often used in groups, e.g. continence care would be assessed at the same time as privacy and dignity.

Each of these areas is divided into specific items (factors) which are considered, to achieve the overall benchmark or standard. Each factor is assessed using the continuous quality cycle.

Continuous quality cycle

The patient focus of each of these areas is maintained by having a service user, carer, or a representative as part of the overall process for comparing the performance of each clinical area in relation to the statement of best practice. This is referred to as the 'comparison group'. Areas then share good practice to ensure an overall high standard.

The full document is available at:
www.dh.gov.uk/publicationspolicyandguidance

Helen Waldock, Health and Social Care Advisory Service

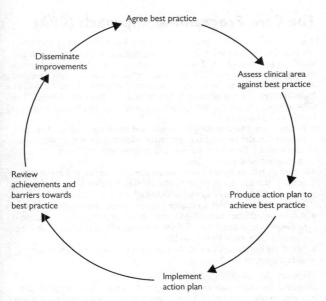

Fig.1.3 Continuous quality cycle.

Further reading

Department of Health. The New NHS: modern, dependable. The Stationery Office: London, 1997.

Department of Health. A first class service: quality in the new NHS. DoH: London, 1998.

Human Rights Act (1998). The Stationery Office: London, 1998. www.hmso.gov.uk/acts

The Essence of Care: Patient focused benchmarking for health care practitioners 2003 DOH London.

The Care Programme Approach (CPA)

The CPA, introduced in 1991, is one of the key processes underpinning the NSF for Mental Health. It is a 'whole systems' (integrated health and social care) approach to clinical effectiveness. The CPA aims to ensure that where possible, the right intervention happens at the right time and in the right place to promote an individual's optimum mental health. Multidisciplinary team working is fundamental to the CPA process. The CPA aims to ensure that the following points of good practice in mental health are adhered to:

- Arrangements for assessing the health and social care needs of people in mental health services are systematic; including a mental state, a risk assessment, a carer's assessment, and a vulnerable children's assessment where applicable.
- A care plan is formulated with the service user; health and social care needs and action to be taken by the services are identified, clarified. and recorded. Where a need is identified and there is no service provision available, this is recorded on an unmet needs register.
- A care coordinator (a qualified mental health professional) is appointed to keep in close touch with the service user, and to monitor their care plan (📖 Case management skills).
- There are regular reviews of the care plan involving the service user and all agencies involved.

There are two levels of CPA:

Standard: for individuals with a recognized mental health problem and a low risk rating, who are able to manage their mental health problem, have supportive social circumstances, and are active participants in their own care. They may require the intervention of one agency or discipline or low-key support from more than one agency or discipline.

Enhanced: for individuals with a recognized mental illness resulting in multiple care needs and requiring multi–agency involvement. They are more likely to have co-existing physical or mental health problems, dis-engage with services and present a higher risk to themselves or others. They will require a higher level and intensity of intervention. Care plans at this level will include a crisis plan.

The CPA is applicable to all people using secondary mental health services regardless of whether they are living at home, are homeless, in hospital, in prison or in residential care. As an individual's mental health needs change, it is possible to move from the standard to enhanced level of CPA and visa-versa. This would be done with involvement from the multidisciplinary team.

Helen Waldock, Health and Social Care Advisory Service

Further reading

Carpenter, J, Sbaraini, S. *Choice, Information and Dignity: involving users and carers in care management in mental health.* The Policy Press: 1997.

NHS and Community Care Act (DoH London). 1990.

The patients charter good practice in mental health services a collection of good practice in the provision of community mental health services 1997. Department of Health, NHS Executive. The Stationary Office London.

Department of Health 2001 An audit pack for monitoring the Care Programme Approach. DoH London.

The Single Assessment Process for older adults (SAP)

The single assessment process was introduced in the NSF for Older People in 2001.[19,20] It aims to ensure that older people's health and social care needs are assessed accurately and at the right time, and that information is not duplicated. There is no particular sequence to the assessment process – the emphasis is on the professional exercising clinical judgment in conjunction with the service user. The aim is that just one professional, where possible, completes and coordinates the assessment. (📖 See Chapter 10 on Older people).

Domains of SAP

All SAP assessments will cover:
- Users perspective; needs, issues, expectations, strengths, and abilities.
- Clinical background; previous conditions, diagnosis, history of falls, and medication use.
- Disease prevention; blood pressure monitoring, nutrition, diet, fluids, vaccination history, alcohol and smoking history, exercise pattern, and screening uptake.
- Personal care and physical well-being; personal hygiene, dressing, pain, oral health, foot health, tissue viability, mobility, elimination, and sleep patterns.
- Senses; sight, hearing, and communication.
- Mental health; cognition, including orientation, memory and dementia, depression, reactions to loss, and emotional difficulties.
- Relationships; social contacts, leisure, hobbies, work, and learning.
- Carer support and strength of caring arrangements; including the carer's perspective.
- Safety; abuse, neglect, fear of crime, and safety in public.
- Immediate environment and resources; care of home and managing daily tasks, such as food preparation, cleaning, and shopping.
  Housing – including, location, access, amenities, heating, and access to local facilities.

Stages in SAP

1) Contact assessment
The initial contact between an older person and a service provider, where significant needs are first described or suspected. Basic personal information is gathered, the nature of the presenting problem is established and the presences of wider health or social care needs are explored.

2) Overview assessment
All or some of the domains identified in the SAP process may be explored, leading to a more rounded assessment and identification of need, deficits, abilities, and strengths.

Helen Waldock, Health and Social Care Advisory Service

3) Specialist assessment
The exploration of a specific need. A specialist assessment will confirm the presence, extent, cause, and likely prognosis of a health or social care condition, for example, a mental health problem. Links may be made to the interactive nature of multiple pathology and social situations.

4) Comprehensive assessment
This can involve pulling together the information gleaned from all stages of the assessment, especially when there has been more than one specialist assessment. Alternatively, it would be completed people who need intensive or prolonged support such as admission to residential care.

5) Care planning
Following assessment, the information is used as the basis for a single plan that addresses all the domains assessed, including the carers assessment. This care plan is then reviewed at regular intervals, at least once a year.

6) Care programme approach (📕 CPA)
Where significant mental health or mental illness needs, such as schizophrenia or dementia are identified, the CPA would be applied. This is outlined in standard 7.5 of the NSF for older people.

References

19 Department of Health. SAP assessment scales. DoH: London, 2003. www.dh.gov.uk
20 Department of Health. National Service Framework for Older People 2001. DoH: London.

Further reading

The Carers and Disabled Children's Act (2000). www.carers.gov.uk DoH London.
Department of Health. The community care assessment directions. DoH: London, 2004. www.dh.gov.uk/policyandguidance
Department of Health. Guidance on the Single Assessment Process for Older People 2002. DoH: London www.dh.gov.uk/publications

The National Service Framework for Mental Health

The National Service Framework for Mental Health (1999) is a long-term strategy, and a landmark in the development of mental health services across England for adults up to the age of 65 years. It clarifies what the National Standards are for service provision and what they aim to achieve. This document directs the changes and modernization needed to bring mental health services into the twenty-first century.

Aims

- Ensure that health and social services promote mental health and reduce discrimination and social exclusion associated with mental health problems.
- Deliver better primary mental health care, and to ensure consistent advice and help for people with mental health needs, including primary care services for individuals with severe mental illness.
- Ensure that each person with severe mental illness receives the range of mental health services they need and that crises are anticipated and prevented where possible.
- Ensure that people in crisis receive prompt and effective help, and timely access to an appropriate and safe mental health place or hospital bed, including a secure bed, as close to home as possible.
- Ensure health and social services assess the needs of carers who provide regular and substantial care for those with severe mental illness, and provide care to meet their needs.
- Ensure that health and social services play their full part in achieving the target of reducing the suicide rate by one fifth by 2010 as directed in 'Saving Lives: our Healthier Nation.'

Standards

All NSF standards are monitored at a local and national level, leading to national performance tables.

Standard 1 – Mental health promotion

- Promote mental health for all, working with individuals and communities.
- Combat discrimination against individuals and groups, and promote their social inclusion.

Standards 2 and 3 – Primary care and access to services

Service users who contact their primary health team with a common mental health problem should:
- Have their mental health needs identified and assessed.
- Be offered effective treatments, including referral to specialist services for further assessment, treatment, and care if they need it.
- Be able to make contact with local mental health services 24 hours a day and receive adequate care.

Helen Waldock, Health and Social Care Advisory Service

- Be able to use NHS Direct for first level advice and referral to specialist help-lines or to local services.

Standards 4 and 5 – Effective services for people with SMI

- Receive care that optimizes engagement and anticipates or prevents a crisis thereby reducing risk.
- Have a copy of their written care plan which:
  a) States the action to be taken in a crisis by the service user, their carer, and their care coordinator.
  b) Advises the GP how they should respond if the service user needs additional help.
  c) Is regularly reviewed by the care coordinator.
  d) Enables them to access services 24 hours a day, 365 days per year.

Service users who are assessed as needing a period of care away from their home should have:
- Timely access to an appropriate hospital bed or place which is:
  a) In the least restrictive environment, and consistent with the need to protect them and the public.
  b) As close to home as possible.
- A copy of a written care plan, agreed on discharge, which sets out their care and rehabilitation, identifies their care coordinator, and specifies the action to be taken in a crisis.

Standard 6 – Caring about carers

All carers or people who provide regular and substantial care for a person on CPA should:
- Have an assessment of their caring, physical and mental health needs repeated on at least an annual basis.
- Have their own written care plan given to them, and implemented with them.

Standard 7 – Preventing suicide (□ Suicide)

Local health and social care services should aim to prevent suicides by:
- Combining all the above standards into a local delivery plan based on local need.

And in addition:
- Support local prison staff in preventing suicides among prisoners.
- Ensure that staffs are competent to assess the risk of suicide among individuals.
- Develop a local system for suicide audit, to learn lessons and take any necessary action.

The full document is available at www.dh.gov.uk.

Further reading

All documents are available in PDF format on the Department of Health (UK) website at www.dh.gov.uk
A First Class Service: Quality in the new NHS, 1998.
Saving Lives: Our Healthier Nation, 1999.
Modernising mental health services, 2002.
The NHS Plan, 2000.
The NHS Plan: a progress report, 2003.

The National Service Framework for Older People

The National Service Framework for Older People was launched in England in 2001. It provides the drive and focus for a ten year strategic development plan of all older peoples services. The framework informs the culture and attitude of all professionals across all disciplines and is recognized as a speciality area in its own right. (📖 See Chapter 10 on Older People).

The Framework has four underlying principles:
• Respecting the individual.
• Intermediate care.
• Providing evidence based specialist care.
• Promoting an active, healthy life.

The aims of the Framework are to:
• Ensure older people are never discriminated against in accessing NHS or social care services as a result of their age.
• Ensure that older people are treated as individuals, and receive appropriate and timely packages of care which meet their needs as individuals, regardless of heath and social care boundaries.
• Provide integrated services to promote faster recovery from illness, prevent unnecessary hospital admissions, support timely discharge, and maximize independent living.
• Ensure older people receive the specialist help they need in hospital and that they receive maximum benefit from having been in hospital. Reduce the incidence of stroke in the population and ensure that after a stroke, people have prompt access to integrated stroke services.
• Reduce the number of falls which result in serious injuries, and ensure effective treatment and rehabilitation afterwards.
• Promote good mental health in older people, and to treat and support those older people with dementia and depression.
• Extend the healthy life expectancy of older people.

Standards

All NSF standards are monitored at a local and national level, leading to national performance tables.

1) Rooting out age discrimination

Services will be provided, regardless of age, on the basis of clinical need alone. Social care services will not use age in their policies or eligibility criteria, to restrict access to available services.

2) Person-centred care

NHS and social care services treat older people as individuals and enable them to make choices about their care. This is achieved through the single assessment process, integrated commissioning arrangements, and integrated provision of services, including community equipment and continence services.

Helen Waldock, Health and Social Care Advisory Service

3) Intermediate care

Older people will have access to a new range of intermediate care services at home, or in designated care settings, to promote their independence. These enhanced services from the NHS and local authorities will aim to prevent unnecessary hospital admissions and will provide effective rehabilitation services to enable early discharge from hospital. They also aim to prevent premature or unnecessary admission to long-term residential care.

4) General hospital care

Older people's care in hospital is delivered through appropriate specialist care and by hospital staff who have the right set of skills to meet their needs.

5) Stroke

The NHS will take action to prevent strokes, working in partnership with other agencies where appropriate.

6) Falls

The NHS, working in partnership with local authorities will take action to prevent falls and as a result, reduce fractures or injuries in their populations of older people.

7) Mental Health in older people

Older people who have mental health problems will have access to integrated mental health services, provided by the NHS and local authorities to ensure effective diagnosis, treatment and support for themselves and their carers.

8) The promotion of health and an active life in older age.

The health and well being of older people is promoted through a co-ordinated programme of action led by the NHS with support from local authorities.

The full document is available at www.dh.gov.uk. Including examples of service models and care pathways.

Further reading

All documents are available on the Department of Health (UK) website at www.dh.gov.uk
Carers and Disabled Childrens' Act, 2000.
National Service Framework for Older People: report of progress and future challenges, 2003.
Keep Well, Keep Warm Campaign, 2004.
National Care Standards Commission (NCSC) up to date information is available at www.csci.org.uk.

The biological context of mental health

Recent years have seen many changes to the provision of services and therapies for people suffering from mental illness, but there is still a slant towards the biological context of mental health.

Historical context

In primitive times, people believed that mental illness was created by evil spirits entering and taking over the body. Their expulsion was facilitated by a healer, medicine man, or spiritualist via magic or reincarnation.

Ancient civilization, notably the Romans, Greeks, and Arabs, believed the mentally ill should be treated humanely, sedated with opium, but with good hygiene, good nutrition, activity, and social occupation. The Greek physician Hippocrates was the first to attempt to classify mental illness. Controversies about the approaches to treatment were apparent ranging from the drilling of a person's skull to let the spirits out, to good counsel (direction and advice).

After the fall of the Roman Empire – around 500–1450 AD – mental illness became surrounded by witchcraft, superstition, magic, and fear. Some were locked away in asylums, some were hidden by their families, while others were left to fend for themselves.

In the 14th–17th centuries the mentally ill were thought to pose a risk to society. They were put in prison or in asylums and were often subject to cruel regimes, such as being locked in cages or chained to walls for containment. The first mental hospital, The Bethlem Royal, was established in the UK. People could visit, and for a small fee observe the inmates.

In the 18th–19th centuries, social changes included urbanization and impoverishment on a large scale. The asylums or madhouses were closely associated with the workhouses, and were presided over by a medical superintendent – despite the awareness of 'moral treatment' (pioneered by William Tuke, where restraint was kept to a minimum and people were engaged in occupational tasks). In 1845 the Lunatics Act was introduced, and the approach to mental illness was consolidated with the introduction of the new sub-specialty of medicine, called Psychiatry. The psychiatrist became the responsible guardian of the lunatic, thus medical doctors sought to improve their knowledge about the cause and treatment of mental illness. At this time a physiological explanation was the most common rationale for mental illness.

In the 20th century the asylum population continued to grow, until in the later half of the 20th century it was decreed that the asylums should close. The introduction of phenothiazines (major tranquilizers) reinforced the position of the psychiatrist as treating mental illness, while attendants and nurses contained the patients. Within the field of psychiatry, interest in the biological causes of mental illness remained dominant, with the introduction of new forms of treatment with fewer side-effects.

Helen Waldock, Health and Social Care Advisory Service

In the 21st century the nature or nurture debate continues. There is now recognition that behaviour is the product of both, with each contributing to the development of mental health and mental illness. There is an increasing evidence base to support non-medical interventions alongside the role of the psychiatrist. The discovery of the genome is likely to bring the greatest advances to psychiatry over the next decade, although how this will impact is not yet known. Medical science continues to dominate in terms of economics, and social status, with more recourses being allocated to medical research and consultants continuing to manage resources (beds), whilst contributing to the care of an individual, although this is gradually being challenged by the growth in the service user movements and the thrust of current mental health policy.

Further reading

Breggin, PR. *Toxic Psychiatry*. Harper Collins: London, 1993.

Lomax, M. *The Experience of an Asylum Doctor*. George Allen & Unwin: 1921 London.

Rogers, A, Pilgrim, D. *Experiencing Psychiatry: Users views of services*. Macmillan: London, 1993.

Rogers, A, Pilgrim, D. *Mental Health Policy in Britain* Palgrave Macmillan UK 2001.

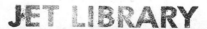

The socio-cultural context of mental health

Sociology refers to the study of the social lives of humans, groups, and societies. It is concerned with social rules and processes that bind and separate people, not only as individuals, but as members of associations, groups, and institutions. It is relevant to today's health care institutions, whether they in a hospital or in a community, as they help us understand how we got to where we are.

Ivan Illich, a well known author of an informal series of controversial critiques of the institutions of 'modern' culture, used the concept of 'iatrogenesis' to describe illnesses caused by medical practice.[21] This concept describes the ways in which the activities of doctors may have harmful results, for example the ill effects of prescribed medication. Another theme of Illich's work is the mis-allocation of resources, where the highest investment is allocated to technology or high prestige medicine such as cardiac surgery, leaving the 'Cinderella services' such as mental health, and care of the elderly suffering. Some would argue that this is still the current situation in the UK. Illich has been criticized for underestimating the advances in modern health care.

Talcott Parsons, a sociologist who attempted to integrate all the social sciences into a science of human action, stressed the importance of health for the smooth running of society.[22] He developed the concept of the 'sick role' involving certain rights and obligations, which should restore the sick person to health as soon as possible (see below). There is much to think about when this is applied to mental health.

Rights and obligations of the 'Sick Role'

Obligations	Rights
Person must wish to recover as soon as possible	Person is relieved of usual responsibilities and tasks
Person must seek professional advice and follow prescribed treatment	Person is accorded sympathy and support

Whilst recognizing that not all illnesses are sufficiently severe enough to fit into the sick role, Parsons describes ways in which society expects an ill person to behave and which can account for society's attitude to those who do not conform.

Inequalities in health

Inequalities in health were first brought into the public domain with the publication of the Black Report in 1980. This showed that the lower the social class you were, the more likely you were to become ill or die prematurely. Whilst the focus was not on mental health, the factors concerning physical health directly impact on mental health; the more economically advantaged you are the better your health and the greater your life chances.

There are three broad types of inequality in mental health:

- Inequality in access to health care, e.g. access of refugees to primary health care or treatment for PTSD (📖 Post-traumatic stress disorder).
- Inequality in heath and health outcomes e.g. there is a 6 year difference in average life expectancy for people living in different London boroughs.
- Inequalities in the determinants of health, access to the means of financial reward: the better educated the more likely you will have a better income therefore better housing, diet, and so on e.g. 70% of those with a psychotic disorder are unemployed.

Different groups and categories of people have very different experiences of the determinants of health. Some are well known, such as gender, age, social class, ethnicity, geographical area. Others such as disability, single parenthood, quality of school, age of housing, type of road user, are less obvious. Inequalities can become entrenched when these categories overlap e.g. a combination of age, ethnic group, and area. In these circumstances, there can be a snowballing effect leading to pockets of deprivation and increased *rates of mental illness, such as are seen in some deprived inner city areas*

References

21 Illich, I. Medical Nemesis: the exploration of health. Calder & Boyars: London, 1957.
22 Parsons, T. The Social System. Routledge: London, 1951.

Further reading

Townsend, P, Davidson, N. *Inequalities in Health – The Black Report.* Penguin: 1986. UK.
The Black Report www.sochealth.co.uk

Mental health promotion

Standard one of the NSF for mental health

Mental health services and staff have a direct interest in promoting positive mental health and well-being in individuals, the family and the work place. Mental health promotion involves any action to enhance the mental well-being of an individual, families, communities, and organizations. It is important to recognize that everyone has mental health needs, whether or not they have a diagnosis of mental illness. Mental health programmes that target the whole community will also benefit those who have mental health problems.

Mental health promotion is essentially concerned with

- How individuals, families, organizations, and communities think and feel.
- The factors that influence how we think and feel, individually and collectively.
- The impact this has on overall well-being.

Mental health promotion works at three levels:

- Strengthening individuals – or increasing emotional resilience through interventions designed to promote self esteem, life and coping skills, relationship and parenting skills.
- Strengthening communities – increasing social inclusion and participation, improving local environments, developing health and social services to support mental health, anti-bullying strategies in schools, work place health, community safety, childcare and self-help networks.
- Reducing structural barriers to mental health – through initiatives to reduce discrimination and inequality by promoting access to education, meaningful employment, housing services, and support for those who are vulnerable.

At each level, interventions may focus on strengthening factors known to protect mental health (e.g. social support, job control) or to reduce factors know to increase risk (e.g. unemployment, violence).

The benefits of mental heath promotion are:

- Improving physical health and well-being.
- Providing capability to cope with mental distress in life.
- Preventing or reducing the risk of mental health problems, notably behavioural disorders, depression and anxiety, substance misuse.
- Assisting recovery from mental health problems.
- Reducing the stigma and discrimination associated with having mental health problems or using mental health services.
- Strengthening the capacity of communities to support social inclusion, tolerance and participation and reducing vulnerability to socio-economic stressors.
- Increasing mental health awareness.
- Improving health at work, increasing productivity and reducing sickness absence.

Helen Waldock, Health and Social Care Advisory Service

Community strategies are usually coordinated by a local strategic partnership including health, primary care, education, transport, voluntary sector, social services, and local government, and are available at local town halls and libraries.

Further reading

MacDonald, T. *The Social Significance of Health Promotion*. Routledge: London, 2003.
Tudor, K. *Mental Health Promotion: paradigms and practice*. Routledge: London, 1996.

Transcultural mental health nursing

Transcultural nursing is a humanistic and scientific area of study. It focuses on differences and similarities among cultures with respect to health and illness. It aims to use knowledge of people's cultural values, beliefs and practices to provide culturally specific or culturally congruent nursing care.

Culture refers to the norms and practices of a particular group that are learned and shared and that guide thinking, decisions, and actions. Cultural values are an individual's desired or preferred way of acting or knowing something, sustained over a period of time, and which govern actions or decisions.

Culturally diverse nursing care is an optimal mode of health care delivery. It refers to the variability of nursing approaches needed to provide culturally appropriate care, incorporating an individual's cultural beliefs, values, and practices.

📖 Culturally capable mental health nursing

It is relevant in the UK because:
• Minority ethnic groups report higher scores of psychological distress.
• Rates of psychotic illness are twice as high in African-Caribbean people than in their white counterparts.
• Ethnic minorities are six times more likely to be detained under the mental health act.
• Women born in East Africa have a 40% higher suicide rate than those born in the UK or Wales.
• Irish people have suicide rates 53% in excess of other minority ethnic groups.

To be culturally competent, the nurse needs to understand their own and their patient's world view, but to avoid stereotyping and misapplying scientific knowledge e.g. *interpretation of somatic symptoms*. Different cultures have different perceptions of illness and disease and their causes, and this affects their approaches to health care. Culture also influences how people seek health care and how they behave towards health care providers. How people are cared for and how they respond to this care is greatly influenced by culture. Health care providers must have the ability and knowledge to communicate with all their patients and to understand health behaviours influenced by culture. This ability and knowledge can reduce barriers to the delivery of health care.

There are five essential elements that contribute to an organization becoming culturally competent:
• Valuing diversity.
• Having the capacity for cultural self-assessment.
• Being conscious of the dynamics inherent when cultures interact.
• Having a workforce that reflects the local population to enhance cultural knowledge.
• Having developed adaptations of service delivery reflecting an understanding of cultural diversity e.g. female only clinics.

Helen Waldock, Health and Social Care Advisory Service

Major challenges to transcultural care include:
- Recognizing clinical differences among people of different ethnic and cultural groups.
- The challenges of communication; working with interpreters, nuances of words in different languages.
- Ethical challenges; while western medicine is the most dominant in the world, it does not have all the answers. Respect for the belief systems of different cultures, and the effects of those beliefs on well-being are crucial.
- The effect of an authority figure is not always apparent; but many people are wary of caregivers. Some may have been victims of atrocities at the hands of authorities in their homelands.

As individuals and caregivers, nurses need to learn to ask questions sensitively and to show respect for different cultural beliefs. More importantly, they must listen carefully to patients.

Further reading

Cross, T, Baxron, B, Dennis, K, Issacs, M. *Towards a Culturally Competent System*, vol. 1. Georgetown University: Washington DC, 1989.
Minarik, PA. *Culture and Nursing: a pocket guide California*. Rittenhouse Book Distributors: 1997.

Models of mental health nursing

Early models of nursing evolved in the context of economic, societal, and technological changes. Today, the systems of health care organization and nursing care delivery continue the challenge of adaptation in a rapidly changing service.

Systems of mental health nursing
- *Functional nursing*; technical tasks are assigned to staff according to the complexity of the task and the knowledge and skill of the nurse.
- *Team nursing*; a team of nurses deliver care to a group of patients who are assigned to each team member according to the complexity of the patients needs. A team leader is accountable for coordinating care and delegating to the team.
- *Primary nursing*; a registered nurse is accountable for the care planning from admission to discharge, promoting continuity, and delegating to an associate nurse as required.
- *Case management*; a collaborative approach with the nurse as the co-ordinator, not necessarily providing direct patient care.

Aspects of all four approaches are used depending on the environment, the work load, and the individual needs of patients.

The nursing process
The nursing process is a systematic, goal-directed, flexible and rational approach to care. It ensures consistent, continuous, quality nursing care and provides a basis for professional accountability. The steps of the nursing process are cyclic, overlapping and interrelated.
1. Assessment (of patient's needs) (📖 Assessment of mental health needs).
2. Diagnosis (of human response needs that nursing can assist with).
3. Planning (of patient's care).
4. Implementation (of care).
5. Evaluation (of the success of the implemented care).

Theories and models of nursing
Nursing models are conceptual models, constructed of theories and concepts. They are used to help nurses assess, plan, and implement patient care by providing a framework within which to work.

There are four concepts or paradigms that are fundamental to all nursing models and theories, these being man, health, environment, and nursing. The relationship between these paradigms is explored with the beliefs of the person writing the theory thereby guiding the focus of the theory. Within mental health, relationships are acknowledged as being the fifth paradigm. There are over forty models of nursing to choose from, and the skill of choosing the right one is to explore the belief and value

Helen Waldock, Health and Social Care Advisory Service

systems underpinning them. In mental heath, the four most commonly used models are:

Imogene King: the general systems framework[23]

King's conceptual framework includes three types of dynamic interacting systems. These are: personal systems (represented by the individual), interpersonal (represented by dyadic interactions), and social systems (represented by broader connections such as the family or health services). This model focuses on goal attainment, acknowledging that each bring their own perceptions and judgements to an interaction.

Dorothea Orem: self-care framework[24]

Orem's model focuses on an individual's ability to perform self-care. Self- care activities vary depending on individual circumstances. Self care requisites can be divided into universal (applicable to all e.g. breathing), developmental (a particular point in life e.g. pregnancy), or health deviation requisites (when unwell). Self-care deficits are identified with the nurse and the patient working together in a wholly compensatory, partially compensatory, or supportive educative system to address the deficits.

Rosemarie Parse: man-living-health[25]

Parse's theory views human beings as an open system. Using three core principles she describes man (generic term) as a unique individual with unique reactions to illness. The nurse's role is to become fluent in the uniqueness of the individual accepting their language, values, beliefs, desires, pace of life and so on, and through practice enable the individual to move forward to live a fulfilled life as determined by themselves.

Hildergard Peplau: the theory of interpersonal relations[26]

The nurse and the patient work together toward solutions for everyday encounters. Peplau identifies four sequential phases in the nurse-patient relationship: orientation, identification, exploitation, and resolution. The nurse fulfils different roles throughout the stages of the relationship, teacher, resource, counsellor, leader, technical expert, and surrogate.

All theories and models have their strengths and weaknesses. It is worth referring to the original texts to get the accurate meaning.

References

23 King, IM. A Theory for Nursing: systems, concepts, process New York. A. Wiley Medical Publications: 1981.

24 Orem, D. Nursing: concepts of practice. Mosby: St Louis, 1995.

25 Parse, R. Man Living Health: A theory of nursing. Wiley: New York, 1981.

26 Peplau, HE. Interpersonal Relations in Nursing. GP Putnam: New York, 1952. Reprinted 1991, Springer: New York.

Mental health nursing in context

From the beginning of time, people with mental health problems, mental disorders, or what was defined as socially deviant behaviour, have received some form of care or control.

From asylum to community

Asylums housed the 'insane' from the 12th century, where they suffered degradation, repression, and cruelty. In the 17th century, the pioneers Philippe Pinnel in France, and William Tuke in the UK introduced reforms unchaining the 'lunatics' and creating havens for the insane. Physical restraints were replaced with moral constraints based on reason, supported by meaningful work, social and recreational activities within a domestic type environment. This marked the beginning of changing attitudes towards the insane.

During the 19th century, the asylums were rapidly expanded, catering for thousands of people, and quickly became overcrowded and custodial in nature, with many allegations of malpractice. County authorities were expected to provide their own asylums, for the care or incarceration of the insane. Private institutions had existed before this, and provided the only care available. Throughout this period, private institutions continued to exist and be founded for so called idiots and imbeciles, who were usually those who today would be said to have learning disabilities. The county asylum structure was nationalized in 1948, when the institutions were absorbed into to the National Health Service

In 1926, a Royal Commission investigated the lunacy laws resulting in the Mental Treatment Act coming into being; it defined categories of voluntary and temporary patients, and by 1959 the Mental Health Act put medical professionals in control, with a strong emphasis on community involvement.

In 1961 the government of the time declared that the asylums must close, and by the 1960s there was a decline in asylum numbers due to:
- Gross overcrowding.
- Deterioration in the fabric of the buildings.
- Increasing labour costs.
- The view that medication could control symptoms.
- The increasing role of the consultant psychiatrist.
- The increased influence of the anti-psychiatry movement.
- Scandals and public enquiries highlighting neglect and suffering.
- Government policy that stated mental hospitals must close and local facilities be developed.

This has remained the approach of all national policy to the current time. Many of the large institutions did not finally close their doors until 1990s.

The 1983 Mental Health Act (currently under review) protects the rights of the detained patient.

From attendants to nurses

All branches of nursing arose under the patronage of the medical profession. Initially, attendants in institutions were there for their personal and moral qualities; they were expected to have physical strength, be sober, set a positive example and offer guidance. For this, they had their meals with the patients, slept in rooms off the wards, and worked 15 hours a day. As a result, many of them became as institutionalized as their charges.

It was not until the late 19th century that consideration was given to the education of the attendants. This came in the form of a handbook from the Royal Medico-Psychological Association (RMPA), known as 'The Instruction of Attendants on the Insane'. This later formed the basis of the first recordable qualification in mental health nursing.

Due to overcrowding in the asylums, bureaucratic nurse patient hierarchies became the norm. These relied on strength and intimidation rather than friendliness and common sense. An uneasy relationship between the general hospital nurses and the attendants began to develop as the governing body, the British Nursing Association (BNA), refused entry to those who had completed their RMPA training on the grounds of social standing, as general nursing was then a middle class occupation.

It was not until the General Nursing Council (GNC) (predecessor to the UKCC and NMC) started its own courses for psychiatric nursing that the attendants were permitted onto the national register. This made little difference to career pathways, as most asylum matrons were general nurses. This has been ameliorated to some extent with the introduction of Project 2000 with the shared common foundation programme.

The decline of the asylums brought changes for nurses. Many of them were resistant to their closure as this was a direct threat to their economic stability. Even in the 1950s, many lived in the grounds of the institution around which their social life revolved.

But this was a time of opportunity; many nurses who believed in their profession moved into innovative roles in the district general hospital psychiatric units, day hospitals, outpatient departments, and after care services. This led to the placement of community psychiatric nurses in primary care, a role that did not survive as government policy was to focus services on those who were deemed SMI, although this is being reversed with the implementation of the NSFMH.

Mental health nursing today

The current government drive towards integrated care and primary mental health care has led to a variety of post registration qualifications, and to the development of a mental health practitioner who does not have to be a registered nurse. Conflict remains within mental health nursing about the future of the profession. This is not just in relation to other branches of nursing, but it relates to the unanswered question of 'do you need to be a mental health nurse to provide mental health care now that there is a move away from the medical model towards a more socially inclusive model?'

Further reading

Goffman, E. *Asylums*. Penguin Books Ltd 1991 London.

McMillan, I. Years of Bedlam Nursing, *Times* **92**(47) 62–3, 20 Nov, 1996.

Nolan, P. *History of Mental Health Nursing*. Nelson Thornes Ltd: 1998 Chetenham UK.

Nolan, P. Annie Altschul's Legacy to British Mental Health Nursing. *Journal of Psychiatric and Mental Health Nursing* **6**(4): 267–72, 1999.

Rehabilitation and recovery

Recovery for each person is an individual journey and therefore unique. At some point in our lives we all need the support of another. Knowing yourself, your own signs and symptoms is an important step to wellness, regardless of whether you have a mental illness or not.

The concept of recovery is having a substantial impact on service users, families, mental health researchers, and service delivery. It was introduced in the writings of service users in the 1980s, who had recovered to the extent of being able to write about their experiences, coping with symptoms, getting better, and gaining an identity.

There is no single definition of recovery, nor a single way to measure it, but the overreaching message is that hope and restoration to a meaningful life are both possible despite a serious mental illness. Recovery does not always mean cure but involves less interference of symptoms in everyday life.

Recovery is different to rehabilitation, which is seen as a specialist service, as opposed to a process or concept. Rehabilitation combines pharmacological and social support to service users and families in order to improve their lives and their functional capacity. Recovery does not refer to any specific service, but to the experience of gaining a new and valued sense of self and purpose.

Principles of recovery:
- It concerns the whole of an individual's life; this includes their relationships, friends, family, housing, money, work, education, social activities and life, medication, and therapies. The CPA provides the framework for this, providing a coordinated approach and using experts where necessary.
- It concerns personal growth and development; assessment should not only consider symptoms and problems, but strengths and abilities. Services need to fit around the user, rather than have the user fit into the services.
- Recovery is ongoing; there is no time limit to support, although this may vary as an individual fluctuates. The role of maintenance support provided by a coordinator or support worker is important – this is a meaningful long-term relationship that may 'hold' a person through a difficult time.
- It concerns the wider context of social inclusion outside mental health services; including meaning in life, work, home relationships, culture, and beliefs. The role of the professionals is to enable access to what people want, empowering individuals to take part in their own lives.
- Access to peer support is seen as valuable; this may be via self-help groups, or voluntary organizations such as Mind. The way forward is via public and patient involvement in designing and delivering services.

Helen Waldock Health and Social Care Advisory Service

The impact of recovery is felt most by users and their families, who are energized by the message of hope and self-determination. Having a more active role in treatment, research, social and vocational functioning, and personal growth strikes a responsive chord in users of services. Harbouring more optimistic attitudes and expectations may improve the course of the illness yet direct empirical evidence to support recovery is still in its infancy.

Further reading

Jacobson, N. *In Recovery: the making of mental health policy*. Vanderbilt University Press: 2004.

Moxley, DP. *Sourcebook of Rehabilitation and Mental Health Practice*. Kluwer Academic Publishing USA: New York 2003.

Newbiggin, K, Wells, A, West, A. *Working for Mental Health*. Health and Social Care Advisory Service: 2004. London.

Essential mental health nursing skills

Mental health assessment

Assessment is an important stage in the nursing care of people with mental health problems. It involves collecting information and using it to decide on the need for, and the nature of, any subsequent mental health care. Assessing people's mental state involves judging their psychological health; this requires experience, a degree of intelligence, self-insight, social skills, objectivity, and the ability to deal with cognitive complexities. A mental health nursing assessment is often done during an assessment interview, but may be an ongoing dynamic process.

Reasons for doing a mental health assessment include:
• Identifying a person's needs.
• Assisting in developing and using appropriate interventions.
• Contributing to diagnostic accuracy.
• Defining a problem that needs solving.

What should be assessed?
📖 The experience of mental illness
• The biological self – (📖 physical health care), should include BMI and urinalysis.
• The behavioural self – how the person thinks, feels, and acts.
• The social self – how people interact with others, family history.
• The spiritual self – the person's hopes, dreams, and beliefs.
• The cultural self – beliefs and morals.
• Past history – of psychiatric disorder and physical health status.
• Current financial, social functioning, and environmental factors e.g. employment, benefits, living arrangements, social activities.
• Psychiatric diagnosis and current symptoms, past and present.
• Appearance and behaviour – physical appearance, reaction to situation.
• Mood – current mood and recent changes.
• Speech – rate, form, volume and quantity of information, content.
• Form of thought – amount and rate of thought, continuity of ideas.
• Thought content – delusions, suicidal thoughts.
• Perception – hallucinations, other perceptual disturbances.
• Cognition – level of consciousness, memory, orientation, concentration, abstract thoughts.
• Insight – understanding of condition.
• Sexual health – sexual activity, contraceptive use, substance use.

The end product of assessment
By the end of the assessment you should be able to:
Measure – the scale and size of needs.
Clarify – the context or conditions under which needs and problems exist.
Explain – the purpose, function, impact, and stability of an individual's behaviour.

Patrick Callaghan, Professor of Mental Health Nursing, University of Nottingham & Nottinghamshire Healthcare NHS Trust

Methods of data collection during assessment

Interviews

Gathering information through questioning. The goal of the interview is to describe, diagnose, and begin the therapeutic relationship. The aims of the interview are to build trust and identify needs.

Rating scales

These are often used with interviews, as part of a mental health assessment. Some commonly used rating scales in mental health assessment are as follows:

- The Short Form-12 (SF-12) – a measure of general mental and physical health.
- The Health of the Nation Outcome Scale (HoNOS) – a measure of 12 categories of behaviour and mental state linked to mental health status.
- Brief Psychiatric Rating Scale (BPRS) – a measure of psychiatric symptoms.
- Beck Depression Inventory (BDI) – a measure of depressive symptoms.
- Side-effects Checklist (SEC) – a measure of side-effects of drugs commonly used in psychiatry.
- Suicide Assessment and Management (SAM) – a measure of suicidal intent and previous self-harming behaviour.
- Social Functioning Scale (SFS) – a measure of day-to-day functioning that can be impaired by mental health problems.
- Carers' Assessment of Managing Index (CAMI) – a measure of stress and coping in people caring for people with mental health problems.

📖 Using rating scales

Further reading

Andrews, G, Jenkins, R (eds.). *Management of Mental Disorders*, UK edn.   Sydney: WHO Collaborating Centre for Mental Health and Substance Misuse, 1999.

Barker, PJ. *Assessment in psychiatric and mental health nursing: in search of the whole person*, Nelson Thornes: Cheltenham, 1997.

Norman, I, Ryrie, I. *The Art and Science of Mental Health Nursing*. Open University Press: Buckingham, 2004.

Physical health assessment

The assessment of a patient's physical health is important because some mental health interventions, such as drugs, may cause physical side-effects. People with mental health problems often have an increased risk of physical health problems, and they can exacerbate mental health problems. Assessing physical health provides a baseline indicator against which future changes in health can be assessed.

Types of assessment

Mini assessment

An overview of the patient's physical health, focusing on airway, breathing, circulation, appearance, level of consciousness, and vital signs. Any recent contact with other health care professionals.

Comprehensive assessment

This involves a detailed assessment of a patient's physical health, risk factors, and medical history.

Focussed assessment

This involves an assessment of a specific condition, problem or an assessment of care e.g. a neurological assessment.

Ongoing assessment

Whereby the patient's physical health status is continuously assessed through regular observation and monitoring.

What is assessed?

During a routine physical health assessment the following are looked at:

Temperature – a Tempa-Dot™ is used. 1 minute for oral, 3 minutes for axilla, or tympanic thermometer (electronic hand held device for measuring the body temperature through the ear, usually recorded after a few seconds). It is recommended that mercury thermometers are not used as they are a potential hazard for cross infection and risk management.

Pulse – the number of beats per minute, the rhythm (regular or irregular) and the volume (how strong it feels) is checked. The pulse can be felt in any artery that passes over the surface of a bone, e.g. radial, femoral, carotid.

Respiration – rate and sounds.

Blood pressure – is vital to ensure the patient's safety. It is measured by a sphygmomanometer and has two values: systolic when the heart contracts and diastolic when the heart relaxes. The normal range for adults is 100/60 to 150/90 depending on age. It varies with age in children.

Mobility – the patient's ability to move freely.

Nutrition – food and fluid intake, dietary habits, electrolyte balance.

Patrick Callaghan, Professor of Mental Health Nursing, University of Nottingham & Nottinghamshire Healthcare NHS Trust

Weight and height – exact measures, body mass index (BMI), measurements against standards for sex and ethnic group.

Personal hygiene – the ability to attend to personal hygiene.

Elimination – frequency and nature of bowel and bladder movements.

Skin integrity – check for bruises, cuts, appearance and elasticity of skin, risk of pressure ulcers, oedema.

Sexual health – sexual activity, contraceptive use, cervical screening, testicular examination, HIV status.

Oral hygiene – halitosis (smell on breath), general state of teeth, gums and mouth.

Self-care ability
Safety – risk of falls, self-neglect, harm from others, self-harm.

Drug and alcohol use – substance use, units of alcohol taken per week.

Health-related behaviours – e.g. exercise, smoking.

Sleep pattern – nature and frequency of sleep.

Examples of physical health assessment tools
Waterlow Pressure Sore Risk Assessment
McMaster Health Index
Piper Fatigue Scale.

Further reading
Dougherty, L, Lister, S. (eds.). *The Royal Marsden Hospital Manual of Clinical Nursing Procedures*, 6th edn. Blackwell Publishing: Oxford, 2004.

Care planning

Following an accurate assessment, the next stage in the care process is care planning. The needs that are identified during the assessment stage form the basis of the care plan. A care plan is a written account of how the patient's needs will be met. A well-designed care plan should involve working in partnership with the patient to agree the desired objectives and identify the actions necessary to achieve these objectives. It should provide a rationale for the agreed action, and outline criteria against which to measure progress towards the objectives.

Setting care plan objectives

It is easier to set and evaluate objectives if they are SMART – specific, measurable, achievable, realistic, and time oriented. If there are several objectives it may be necessary to prioritize them – and this should be agreed, where possible, with the patient. Each objective may be part of the achievement of a longer-term goal; it may be useful to state the long-term goal first.

An example of a SMART objective with action designed to achieve the objective, and a proposed evaluation of progress, is shown in the table below, using the fictional character of David. He has recently been unable to attend work because he is unhappy, he prefers to stay in bed most of the day, and is neglecting his personal hygiene. As a result he is very distressed.

Long-term goal: David will return to full-time work within 6 months.

Need	Objective	Action	Rationale	Evaluation
David needs to get out of bed each day and have a shower.	David will be able to get out of bed each day for 5 days, and take a shower.	David will set his alarm for 9am each day.	By setting the alarm, David will be reminded of his objective to get out of bed and take a shower.	By the end of 5 days David will have got out of bed each day and taken a shower.

Tips in care planning
• Work in partnership with the patient where possible.
• Use non-judgemental, user-friendly language.
• Use statements that will have meaning for the patient.
• Set measurable and achievable goals.
• Always indicate a date for evaluation/review.
• Make it clear exactly what action is required and by whom.

Patrick Callaghan Professor of Mental Health Nursing, University of Nottingham & Nottinghamshire Healthcare NHS Trust

Assessing the quality of nursing care plans: Evaluation of Nursing Documentation Schedule (ENDS)[1]

The ENDS is a device for assessing the quality of nursing care plans. The ENDS has five sections pertaining to different parts of the care plan: Assessment, Planning, Problem Identification and Objective Setting, Evaluation, and Discharge Planning. The ENDS has 40 questions, the answers to which determine an overall score indicating the quality of the care plan.

Reference
1 Thomas, BL. The Improvement of Care Planning Documentation in Acute Psychiatric Care. Unpublished PhD Thesis, University of London, 2003

Further reading
Gega, L. Problems, goals and care planning. In: I Norman, I Ryrie (eds.) *The Art and Science of Mental Health Nursing: A Textbook of Principles and Practice.* Open University Press: Buckingham, 2004: pp. 665–78.

Psychosocial interventions with individuals

Psychosocial interventions (PSI) have been developed for people with serious mental illness. They are offered as part of a comprehensive care package that usually includes medication.

Definition

The term psychosocial intervention describes a number of interventions for psychosis that are based on psychological principles, but also address the individual's social context. These include evidence-based interventions such as assessment, psychological management of symptoms, and medication management.

Aim

The overall aim is to reduce the distress associated with symptoms by improving the person's ability to cope, and thereby promoting recovery.

Models

Two key models inform psychosocial interventions:
- *The stress-vulnerability model of psychosis* describes how stress impacts on psychotic symptoms.
- *The cognitive behavioural model* informs the psychological management of symptoms.

Engagement and assessment

Engagement is the process of developing a working relationship by addressing issues that the patient identifies as important.

Assessment focuses on strengths as well as problems, and uses these to develop coping strategies and interventions.

Validated assessment tools are used to assess areas such as mental state, psychotic symptoms, social functioning, and the side-effects of medication. The identification of symptoms such as anxiety or depression will need further assessment.

Formulation

Formulation considers the relationship between symptoms and problems. For example, is anxiety the result of hearing voices or does feeling anxious lead to hearing voices?

The relationship between experiences is not always clear, and it is important not to rush the assessment stage.

Madeline O'Carroll, City University, London

Coping strategies

Nurses can use a range of interventions to help people cope with symptoms, for example, using a personal stereo or MP3 player to drown out voices is a pragmatic intervention. Coping strategy enhancement is a highly structured intervention that involves a detailed analysis of strategies currently being used, and replacing or adding other strategies in a systematic manner.

Psycho-education

This includes exploring beliefs about the nature of schizophrenia using the stress vulnerability model as a guide.

Psychological management of symptoms

A form of cognitive behavioural therapy is used to modify symptoms including hallucinations and delusions.

Further reading

Gamble, C, Curthoys, J. Psychosocial interventions In: I Norman, I Ryrie (eds.) *The Art and Science of Mental Health Nursing: A Textbook of Principles and Practice.* Open University Press: Buckingham, 2004: pp. 265–300.

Psychosocial interventions with families

Family interventions were developed for work with families of people with schizophrenia. A significant body of evidence supporting this work has been developed over forty years; although some services have been slow to offer family interventions.

Families play an important role in supporting and caring for people experiencing psychosis. Often they do this with little or no support from professionals.

Definitions

The term 'family' is used loosely, to refer to relatives, partners, carers, or people who are significant to an individual experiencing psychosis. In some cases this might include staff, such as hostel workers.

Family interventions include education, communication, and problem solving and draw on behavioural and cognitive behavioural models. They aim to reduce the risk of relapse as well as provide support to families.

Working with families

It is recommended that two members of staff work with a family. This enables the modelling of good communication. Sessions are offered in the family home, as this makes it easier for family members to attend.

Assessment

Each member of the family is assessed in relation to their understanding of the causes, symptoms and treatment of psychosis. Some families have limited understanding of these issues; and identifying their beliefs is an important part of the process.

Education and information

The findings from assessment are used to tailor specific educational sessions, so that families are not given information with which they are already familiar. Information can be provided through leaflets that the families are asked to read, and followed up by discussion.

Communication

Good communication can help to reduce stress, and improve problem solving. Ground rules are set regarding communication within sessions, such as members speaking directly to each other, rather than talking about each other, and taking it in turns to speak. Family members are encouraged to praise and support each other, with the aim of building a more supportive emotional climate.

Problem solving

Family workers discuss the steps that make up a problem-solving approach, such as being specific about the problem, identifying solutions, setting goals, and reviewing the outcome.

Madeline O'Carroll, City University, London

Further reading

Kuipers, E, Leff, J, Lam, D. *Family Work for Schizophrenia: a practical guide*, 2nd edn. Gaskell: London, 2002.

Working in groups

The therapeutic work of mental health nurses is often done in groups. Groups have advantages in that they are often time and cost-effective, and can provide multiple sources of feedback. This chapter outlines how nurses can work effectively in groups.

Factors that influence the successful running of groups

Trust – people are more likely to participate in a group if they trust the group process and feel safe in sharing information with others in the group.

Cohesion – a group is cohesive when all members share a common therapeutic goal.

Group roles – the roles and functions that people take in groups may be assigned or adopted by group members. These include: task roles such as information giver; maintenance roles such as encourager, compromiser; and self-serving roles like blocker or aggressor.

Power and influence – this is the process whereby group members influence, or are influenced by others, through the exercise of power.

Stages in forming and running a group

Selecting members

Agreeing ground rules, a group contract and terms of reference e.g. goals, time, length, and frequency of meetings, location, start and end dates, addition of new members, attendance, confidentiality, member interaction outside the group, role of group facilitator and participants, and where necessary, fees and expenses.

Facilitating the group

Skills in facilitating groups include: ensuring adherence to ground rules, encouraging and enabling member's participation, fostering an atmosphere of open discussion, setting boundaries, confronting people who may be assuming self-serving roles or acting in a manner that is harmful to the group.

Ending the group

Bringing the group to a close in a manner that does not leave unresolved tensions, and applying consistency in starting and ending on time.

Factors that could inhibit the success of a group

- Absenteeism
- Incapacitating anxiety
- Failure to end as agreed
- Lack of containment of difficult issues
- Hostility
- Failure to facilitate hope
- Dependence

Patrick Callaghan, Professor of Mental Health Nursing, University of Nottingham & Nottinghamshire Healthcare NHS Trust

- Group members forming into small cliques
- Group members projecting ideas and behaviours onto others
- Focusing on issues external to the group
- Rivalry
- Substance use
- Self-harming behaviours
- Regression i.e. adult members behaving in a child-like manner.

The effectiveness of groups

There is evidence from well-designed studies that group therapy leads to successful outcomes for people living with mental health problems including depression, anorexia nervosa, schizophrenia, alcohol dependency, and suicidal adolescents.

Further reading

Kneisl, CR, Wilson, HS, Trigoboff, E. *Contemporary Psychiatric Mental Health Nursing*. Pearson Prentice Hall: New Jersey, 2004: pp. 683–97.
Roth, A, Fonagy, P. *What Works for Whom? A critical review of psychotherapy research*, 2nd edn. The Guildford Press: New York, 2004.

Working with users and carers

The involvement of service users and carers in mental health nursing is an increasingly important – and audited – measure of quality.

Why involve service users and their carers?

The reasons for involving service users and carers are well understood, and include:

- **The moral imperative** – as citizens and 'owners' of the NHS, service users and carers are entitled to have a voice in all aspects of their health care.
- **Quality improvement** – involvement of service users and carers in education (and research) can lead to deeper clinical insight, resulting in changed attitudes and an improvement in delivered care.
- **The political impetus** – there is a policy drive towards the inclusion of these 'experts through experience' in many aspects of health and social care.

Best practice

Best practice in service user and carer involvement is:

- Cooperative – working in partnership as equals.
- Comprehensive – across all components of education.
- Effective – ensuring meaningful change.
- Ongoing – across the lifespan of the programme.
- Inclusive – representative of all stakeholders.
- Reflexive – critically considering its own ongoing work.

Best practice also includes health care professionals valuing the experience of service users, and recruiting service users into education and training.

The nature of user and carer involvement

In practice, involvement may range from consultation, through collaboration, to service user and carer control.

Consultation

Service users and carers are consulted with no sharing of power in decision-making, although their views may influence the outcome.

Collaboration

An active partnership of service users and carers in the educational process and decision-making.

User and carer control

Service users and carers have overall control, although there is a valid place for professional involvement.

Cooperation and continued input are more likely to occur if service users feel that their contribution is valued; implementation of an involvement strategy is more likely to be successful if it is actively driven and supported by management.

Ian Light, (deceased) formerly City University London

Practical considerations

Remuneration

Payment for time and expertise (with reimbursement for all expenses) is considered best practice. However, the practicalities may be difficult, not least because payment may impact adversely on benefit payments. A useful starting point is *A Fair Day's Pay* by The Mental Health Foundation (www.mentalhealth.org.uk).

Clarity

It may be helpful for active user and carer contributors to have an explicit 'job description' to clarify their responsibilities and commitments.

Support

As well as psychological support, practical support is important – such as facilities for people with special needs, access to facilities, taking into account replacement carer costs, etc.

Effectiveness

It is important to assess the impact of the user and carer's involvement in practice.

Further reading

James, L, Morris, N. *Good Practice Guide: Involving Service Users and Carers in Local Implementation Teams (LITs).* NWMDHC: Manchester, 2001: Foreword.

Simpson, EL, House, AO, Barkham, M. *A Guide to Involving Users, Ex-Users and Carers in Mental Health Service Planning, Delivery or Research: A Health Technology Approach,* Academic Unit of Psychiatry and Behavioural Services, University of Leeds: Leeds, 2002.

Engaging users and carers

Mental health nurses should be working in partnership with users and carers in the delivery of mental health nursing. The relationship between users, carers and practitioners is fluid; it could be one of collaboration with users and carers, consultation with users and carers or a user-led approach.

Getting users and carers involved

Tokenism

Tokenism should be guarded against – it is not cost effective and it impacts negatively on individuals and their constituencies. The extent to which any initiative is felt to be tokenistic should be under continual review.

Representation and diversity

The 'representativeness' of service users and carers is often questioned. While absolute representativeness is not achievable (even with respect to lecturers or researchers), working solutions can be found. An important principle is accessing a diverse local set of service users and their carers.

The 'professionalized' user

There is risk that certain groups or individuals will be 'overused'. A useful approach is for new people to be consistently and regularly approached and recruited.

Approaching users and carers

Attention should be paid to local need and the structure of individual service provision. A useful example is 'Ask the Experts', from the Community Care Needs Assessment Project (CCNAP – see Further reading). Care needs to be taken to include groups who have previously been marginalized, e.g. by ethnicity.

Engaging users and carers

- **Introductions** – check the person's name, introduce yourself, state what your role is, the aim of the interaction and the time allotted.
- **Use non-verbal skills** – such as suitable posture, eye contact, facial expression, tone of voice.
- **Listen actively** – avoid interruption, pay attention, be non-judgemental, do not give direct advice, clarify anything that is unclear, provide enough time, do not undermine the person's problem.
- **Use verbal skills** – paraphrase, that is, repeat back to the person what they have said, reflect on the feelings that may underpin any verbal statement, be empathic and convey your understanding of the impact of what the person is saying.

Ian Light, (deceased) formerly City University London

- *Protect confidential information* – however, be mindful that you will need to breach confidentiality if it is in the person's or in the public's interest to do so, on the grounds that there may be harm to the person or others. The NMC Code of Professional Conduct (📖 chapter 1) provides guidance on this issue. For child protection issues check the Department of Health Guidelines on www.dh.gov.uk

Core attitudes and values for work with users and carers
- Communicate respect
- Communicate empathy
- Communicate genuineness

Setting clinical boundaries
Behaviours – do not give presents, make sexual contact or communicate in a sexual manner, or reveal highly personal information about yourself.
Language – Profanities or swear words should be avoided by both user and nurse.
Touch – Avoid any touching beyond a handshake.

Further reading
Website: http://www.ccnap.org.uk Community Care Needs Assessment Project (CCNAP).

Developing, maintaining, and ending therapeutic alliances

Mental health nursing is based on forming therapeutic relationships between nurses and service users.

Core attitudes and values in working with users and carers[2]

- Communicate respect
- Communicate empathy (📖 Empathy)
- Communicate genuineness.

Developing a therapeutic alliance[2]

- Check the person's name and how they like to be addressed
- Introduce yourself
- State your role
- State the aim of the interaction
- State the time allotted
- Agree ground rules for acceptable and unacceptable behaviours (see below).

Setting clinical boundaries[2]

- **Behaviour** – do not give presents, make sexual contact or communicate in a sexual manner, or reveal highly personal information about yourself.
- **Language** – profanities or swearwords should be avoided by both the service user and the nurse.
- **Touch** – avoid any touching beyond a handshake.
- **Space** – the health care setting is usually the most appropriate place to meet. If you work with the person in another setting, be mindful of safety issues, and the need to respect the fact that you are a guest.

Maintaining the therapeutic alliance[2]

- **Use non-verbal skills** – such as a suitable posture, eye contact, facial expression, or tone of voice.
- **Listen actively** – pay attention, do not interrupt, be non-judgemental, do not give direct advice, clarify anything that is not clear, provide enough time, do not undermine the person's problem.
- **Use verbal skills** – paraphrase i.e. repeat back to the person what they have said, reflect on the feelings that may underpin any verbal statement, be empathic and convey your understanding of the impact of what the person is saying.
- **Protect confidential information** – but be mindful that you will need to breach confidentiality if it is in the person's or the public's interest to do so, if there may be harm to the person or others. The NMC Code of Professional Conduct (📖 Chapter 1 on the Mental Health Act) provides guidance on this issue. For child protection issues check the Department of Health Guidelines on www.dh.gov.uk .

Patrick Callaghan, Professor of Mental Health Nursing, University of Nottingham & Nottinghamshire Healthcare NHS Trust

Ending the therapeutic alliance
- Prepare the person for the end of the alliance.
- End the alliance in a manner that does not leave unresolved tensions or problems.
- End when the goals agreed at the beginning have been achieved.
- Leave the person feeling optimistic and hopeful.

Reference
2 Myles, P, Richards, D. Clinical Skills for Primary Care Mental Health Practice. In: *Primary Care Mental Health* [CD-Rom 3]. Centre for Clinical and Academic Workforce Innovation, University of Lincoln: Lincoln, 2006

Further reading
Nursing and Midwifery Council. Too much information: When to tell and what not to tell your patients. NMC News: London, July 2004.

Empathy

Empathy is a therapeutic response that shows a service user that you understand what they are going through, without needing to go through it yourself.

Empathy involves

- Understanding a person's perception of their experiences.
- Accepting how the person sees him or herself.
- Understanding and validating the person's experience.
- Examining the meaning of what the person says and the feelings he or she is conveying.
- Communicating your understanding verbally so that person can confirm or alter your perceptions.
- Communicating your sensitivity of the person's experience.

Examples of empathic responses

'That must have been difficult for you.'
'It seems that you found that experience quite traumatic.'
'It could not have been easy to go through that.'

The purpose of empathy[3]

- It demonstrates care and understanding.
- If you form inaccurate impressions of someone, they can correct you.
- It helps to focus the discussion onto what is important.
- It enables people to share their experiences with you.
- It minimizes misunderstandings, prejudice and negative assumptions.
- It promotes therapeutic alliances.

Five levels of empathy[3]

- **Inaccurate reflection** – e.g. conveying sympathy, being judgemental.
- **Correcting your misunderstandings** – e.g. understanding the feelings associated with the person's experience.
- **Expressing understanding by communicating empathic responses** – see above.
- **Enhancing the person's understanding** – enabling them to improve their own awareness and insight.
- **Insight** – demonstrating a high level of insight of the meaning of the person's experiences.

Active listening and empathy[4]

Empathy requires the activity to actively listen.
An active listener:

- Does not interrupt.
- Pays attention.
- Is non-judgemental.
- Does not give direct advice.
- Clarifies anything that is unclear.
- Allows adequate time.
- Does not undermine the person's problem.

Patrick Callaghan, Professor of Mental Health Nursing, University of Nottingham & Nottinghamshire Healthcare NHS Trust

References

3 Website: http:// www.mentalhelp.net
4 Myles, P, Richards, D. Clinical Skills for Primary Care Mental Health Practice. In: *Primary Care Mental Health* [CD-Rom 3]. Centre for Clinical and Academic Workforce Innovation, University of Lincoln: Lincoln, 2006.

Further reading

Corazza, E. Empathy, Imagination and Reports. In: *Reflecting the Mind Indexicality and Quasi-Indexicality*. Oxford University Press: Oxford, 2004.

Interpersonal communication

Interpersonal communication is an interaction between people in which they convey their thoughts, feelings, emotions, and behaviour.

The functions of interpersonal communication

(see www.abacon.com)
- To gain information.
- To transmit information.
- To develop your understanding of something.
- To establish your identity role.
- To convey meaning.
- To express your needs.
- To control others.
- To stimulate yourself and relieve boredom.

Forms of interpersonal communication[5]

Non-verbal – this involves posture, personal space preference, eye contact, facial expression, tone of voice, voice quality.

Verbal – this involves paraphrasing or repeating back to the person what they have said, reflecting on the feelings that may underpin any verbal statement, and being empathic by conveying your understanding of the impact of what the person is saying.

Ways to improve your interpersonal communication skills

Listen actively (📖 Engaging users and carers)
- Convey empathy
- Use non-verbal and verbal techniques (see above)
- Practice the skills
- Solicit feedback from others.

Patrick Callaghan, Professor of Mental Health Nursing, University of Nottingham & Nottinghamshire Healthcare NHS Trust

Reference

5 Myles, P, Richards, D. Clinical Skills for Primary Care Mental Health Practice. In: *Primary Care Mental Health* [CD-Rom 3]. Centre for Clinical and Academic Workforce Innovation, University of Lincoln: Lincoln, 2006.

Counselling

Counselling is a form of therapeutic communication designed to enable people to recover from distressing mental health experiences. It should be routinely considered as an option when assessing mental health problems, but is not recommended as the main intervention for severe and complex mental health problems such as personality disorder.

There are many forms of counselling, and each one comes from a different therapeutic tradition. In this chapter we will focus on Cognitive Behavioural and Humanistic counselling.

Cognitive behaviour therapy (CBT)
How effective is CBT?
- CBT was superior to befriending, especially in the long term in people with persistent symptoms of schizophrenia, which are resistant to medication.
- CBT plus standard care was better than standard care alone in reducing relapse rates in people living with schizophrenia.
- CBT significantly benefits physical functioning in adult outpatients with chronic fatigue syndrome (CFS) when compared with relaxation or medical management.
- CBT is beneficial for anxiety disorders, phobias, OCD, chronic pain, PTSD, depression, and chronic fatigue.

Humanistic therapy (HT)
What is HT?
Humanistic therapy derives from humanistic psychology, the so-called 'third force' in psychology (after psychoanalysis and behaviourism).
HT is based on a set of four basic principles:
- The experiencing person is of primary interest.
- Human choice, creativity, and self-actualization are the preferred topics 2° of investigation.
- Meaningfulness must precede objectivity in the selection of research problems.
- Ultimate value is placed on the dignity of the person.

There are different forms of humanistic therapy, but most emphasize the person's natural tendency towards growth and self-actualization. Psychological disorders arise from blocks to the person's attempts to reach their potential. These blocks may be imposed by others who want us to lead lives directed by them. The goal of humanistic therapy is to enable the person to arrive at their own solutions to problems.

It is believed that the main qualities of the humanistic or client-centered therapist are warmth, empathy, and genuineness. The term 'unconditional positive regard' has been used to reflect the therapist's stance.

Patrick Callaghan, Professor of Mental Health Nursing, University of Nottingham & Nottinghamshire Healthcare NHS Trust

The process of HT

Assessment	Treatment	Evaluation
• Identify need/wants of HT • No diagnosis • Initiate mutual decision making • Assessment could create dichotomy	• Working with awareness • Carrying forward • Promoting 7 stages of change	• Level of awareness • Goals achieved • Problem solving ability • Level of coping • Progress towards self-actualization

Indications for HT

Like CBT, HT has been applied to a range of health problems. HT is probably best suited to those who are ready and willing to engage in therapy, who are interested in their inner experience, and who have good social skills and a high need for intimacy.

How effective is HT?

• HT was better than no treatment or waiting list controls, the average client would move from the 50th to the 90th percentile when compared with a pre-therapy sample.
• HT produced more favourable outcomes in clients with relationship problems, anxiety or depression; it produced less favourable outcomes in clients with chronic or more severe problems, like schizophrenia.

Further reading

Department of Health. Treatment choice in psychological therapies and counselling. DoH: London, 2001.

Jones, C, Cormac, I, Mota, J, Campbell, C. Cognitive behaviour therapy for schizophrenia (Cochrane Review). In: *The Cochrane Library*, issue 2. Update Software: Oxford, 2000.

Medication management

Medication for mental health problems should be part of a package of care. Helping clients to manage their prescribed medication is essential to ensure that the maximum benefits of treatments are realized. There is compelling evidence that psychiatric medications are effective in reducing the distress associated with symptoms; but taking medication for a sustained period is difficult for service users. About half of all users will stop taking medication in the first year, resulting in a poorer outcome.

A variety of factors influence whether or not medication is taken regularly. The process of managing medication should be a collaboration between the client and the professional, aiming to remove barriers to adherence and maximize the positive effects of treatment. A process of assessment and intervention should follow.

Assessment

Psychopathology – irrespective of the type of psychiatric medication prescribed, an assessment should be carried out to provide a baseline measurement of symptoms. This assessment should be repeated at relevant intervals to provide a quantitative measure of change and to measure the durability of improvements.

Side-effects of medication – all medications cause side-effects and if these are distressing, the client will find taking it very difficult. An assessment of side-effects is required to identify those that require intervention. Repeated measurement identifies any improvements.

Client's views of treatment – a client's ideas about medication will influence how they will engage in treatment. An assessment of ambivalence can indicate the need for intervention (see below).

Useful assessments include
• Liverpool University Neuroleptic Rating Scale – LUNSERS
• Satisfaction With Antipsychotic Medication Scale – SWAM

Interventions

Side-effects – distressing side-effects should be reduced or eliminated. The appropriateness of the prescription should be evaluated in line with prescribing guidelines. Dose rescheduling to reduce the impact of side-effects can be beneficial, as can practical advice such as early exercise and healthy eating to reduce the likelihood of weight gain.

Exploring views about treatment – everybody has some ambivalence about whether or not to take medication, and this uncertainty is apparent in people who take psychiatric medication. The good things and the not so good things about taking medication can be explored with the client. The good things and the not so good things about stopping medication should also be explored. This approach helps the client to examine their personal beliefs, and it can help to reinforce the belief that the benefits of taking medication outweigh the costs.

Dr Richard Gray & Dan Bressington, Institute of Psychiatry, Kings College, London

Further reading

Gray, R, Bressington, D. Pharmacological interventions and ECT. In: I Norman, I Ryrie (eds.) *The Art and Science of Mental Health Nursing: A Textbook of Principles and Practice.* Open University Press: Buckingham, 2004: pp. 306–28.

Nose, M, Barbui, C, Gray, R, Tansella, M. Meta-analysis of clinical interventions for reducing treatment non-adherence in psychosis. *British Journal of Psychiatry* **183**: 197–206, 2003.

Safe and effective observation of patients

The observation of patients at risk is a key component of psychiatric inpatient nursing care. It is a commonly used nursing intervention for patients 'at risk', and involves the allocation of one nurse (or sometimes two) to one patient for a prescribed length of time, in order to provide intensive nursing care.

Definition

According to the SNMAC practice guidance: Safe and Supportive Observation of Patients at Risk[6], observation is defined as:

'regarding the patient attentively while minimizing the extent to which they feel that they are under surveillance' (p. 12)

Purpose of observation

The main purpose of observation is to keep people safe when they are acutely mentally ill and disturbed. This is especially important for patients who are assessed to be at risk of harming themselves or others, or at risk of being harmed or exploited by others.

Observation is typically used for patients who are:

- Suicidal or actively interested in harming themselves
- Aggressive and who pose a danger to staff or other patients
- Vulnerable
- Prone to abscond
- Sexually disinhibited.

Terminology of observation

There is no universal term to describe observation. The procedure is known by several different terms, for example: special, close, maximum, continuous or constant observation, attention or supervision; suicide watch or precaution; 15 minute or intermittent checks; specialling; one-to-one nursing; nursing observation; and formal observation.

Conducting observation

Observation is generally carried out according to different prescribed levels, which vary in intensity according to the degree of perceived risk. Patients assessed to be at greatest risk of harming themselves or others are nursed on the highest level of observation, with patients never being left alone, and the nurse often within 'arms reach' of the patient. The challenge for nurses who conduct observation is to maintain the safety of 'high risk' patients, whilst maintaining their dignity, privacy, and autonomy.

The decision-making process

Decisions about observation should be made jointly, by the multidisciplinary team. Decisions should be based upon an assessment of risk, using an evidence-based risk assessment tool, consideration of the

Dr Julia Jones, City University, London

patient's history and an interview with the patient and their carer or advocate (as requested by the patient).

Involving the patients and carers in observation

Every effort should be made to involve patients and their carers/friends in the decision-making process, making certain that the procedure of observation and the reasons for its implementation are clearly explained, and ensuring that the observation is conducted in a way that is both supportive and therapeutic.

Reference

6 Department of Health. Practice Guidance: Safe and Supportive Observation of Patients at Risk. In: *Mental Health Nursing: 'Addressing Acute Concerns'*. HMSO: London, 1999.

Further reading

Department of Health. A National Service Framework for Mental Health, HMSO: London, 1999.

Observations of vital signs

Patient observations are an important part of nursing care. They allow the patient's progress to be monitored, and they also ensure prompt detection of adverse events or delayed recovery. Patient observations, or vital signs, traditionally consist of blood pressure, temperature, pulse rate, and respiratory rate. These signs may be observed, measured, and monitored to assess an individual's level of physical functioning. Normal vital signs change with age, sex, weight, and exercise tolerance.

Temperature

Temperature can be measured in many locations on the body. The mouth, ear, axilla, or rectum are the most commonly used places. Temperature can also be measured on the forehead.

Most people think of a 'normal' body temperature as an oral temperature of 37°C. This is an average of a range of normal body temperatures. A person's actual temperature may be 0.6°C above or below 37°C. Normal body temperature changes by as much as 0.6°C throughout the day, depending on activity levels. A rectal or ear (tympanic membrane) temperature reading is 0.3 to 0.6°C higher than an oral temperature reading. A temperature taken in the armpit is 0.3 to 0.6°C lower than an oral temperature reading.

Body temperature is checked to:
• Detect fever (above 37.8°C oral, 38.3°C ear or rectal).
• Detect abnormally low body temperature (hypothermia) in people who have been exposed to cold, shock, alcohol or drug misuse, or infection in frail or elderly people.
• Detect abnormally high body temperature (hyperthermia) in people who have been exposed to heat, causing severe dehydration leading to confusion and delirium.
• Help monitor the effectiveness of a fever-reducing medication.

Respiration

Normal respiration is 15–20 breaths per minute on average. Respiration will vary according to activity level, emotional state, and the use of illicit substances.

Pulse

A normal pulse is 60–80 beats per minute (bpm) at rest. The normal pulse for an adult male is about 72bmp. For an adult female it is 76–80bpm, and 50–65bpm for an elderly person.

Blood pressure

Blood pressure is determined by the amount of blood your heart pumps around your body and the amount of resistance to this blood flow in your arteries. Blood pressure normally varies during the day. It is continually changing, depending on activity, temperature, diet, emotional state, posture, physical state, and medication use.

Helen Waldock, Health and Social Care Advisory Service

Blood pressure readings

Blood pressure readings are usually given as two numbers: for example, 110 over 70 (written as 110/70). The first number is the systolic blood pressure reading; this represents the maximum pressure exerted when the heart contracts. The second number is the diastolic blood pressure reading. This represents the pressure in the arteries when the heart is at rest. The 'average' blood pressure increases from 120/70 to 150/90 with age.

Procedure for taking blood pressure

- The patient should be seated, have rested for 5 minutes and have their arm supported at heart level.
- An appropriate cuff size should be used, and the bladder should nearly (at least 80%) or completely encircle the arm.
- Patients should not have smoked or ingested caffeine within 30 minutes of measurements being taken.
- Measurements should be taken with a mercury sphygmomanometer, a recently calibrated aneroid manometer, or a calibrated electronic device.
- Both systolic and diastolic blood pressure should be recorded.
- Korotkoff's phase V (disappearance of sound) should be used for the diastolic reading.

Maintaining a safe environment

People using mental health services should feel:

Safe – free from harm or abuse – from self or others.

Secure – emotionally safe and secure in that their needs are being met through therapeutic relationships.

Supported – access to staff who connect with them, show them genuine regard, promote their well-being and provide sanctuary.

Essence of care benchmarks for best practice in maintaining safety

Factor	Benchmark for best practice
Orientation to the health environment	All users are fully orientated
Assessment of risk to self	All users have a comprehensive, ongoing assessment of risk to self with involvement of client and significant others
Assessment of risk to others	All users have a comprehensive, ongoing assessment of risk to others with involvement of client and significant others
Balancing observation and privacy in a safe environment	Users are cared for in an environment that balances safe observation and privacy
Meeting clients' safety needs	Users are regularly and actively involved in identifying care that meets their safety needs
A positive culture to learn from complaints and adverse incidents	There is a no-blame culture which allows a vigorous investigation of complaints and adverse incidents and near misses and ensures that lessons are learnt and acted upon

The role of the mental health nurse

The mental health nurse helps to maintain a safe environment for the user by:

- Orientating the user to the environment.
- Working with the user to assess any risk to self and others.
- Identifying safety risks and taking immediate action to remove those risks.
- Setting SMART (Specific, Measurable, Achievable, Realistic, and Time-oriented) care plan objectives to maintain and promote the safety and well-being of users.
- Carrying out agreed interventions to ensure the safety of users and others at all times.

Patrick Callaghan Professor of Mental Health Nursing, University of Nottingham & Nottinghamshire Healthcare NHS Trust

- Reviewing the care plan at agreed intervals to ensure that objectives are being met.
- Modifying the care plan where required, to ensure that objectives are maintaining the user's safety and well being.
- Keeping accurate written records of care provided, to maintain the user's safety and well-being.

Further reading

Department of Health. Essence of Care: patient-focused benchmarking for health care practitioners. DoH: London, 2001.

Department of Health. Safety First: five-year report of the national confidential inquiry into suicide and homicide by people with mental illness. DoH: London, 2001.

Presenting reports of work with users at multidisciplinary meetings and case conferences

Mental health nurses are often called upon to present reports of their work with users in multidisciplinary meetings such as ward rounds and case conferences.

Common features of all reports
- They present facts based on evidence.
- Information provided can be checked and verified.
- Information should be presented in a useful manner.
- They are usually targeted at those with a specific interest in the topic.

Preparing and writing reports
- Gather the information that is required in a systematic manner.
- Use information from as many sources as is needed for a comprehensive and accurate report.
- Work in partnership with users and their significant others in compiling a report.
- Be factual and precise.
- Avoid abbreviations that will not be readily understood by others.
- Avoid jargon and gobbledygook.
- Avoid irrelevant speculation.
- Avoid offensive subjective statements.
- Write in way that can be easily understood.
- Use evidence and/or examples to support statements or judgements.
- Use examples to clarify or illustrate the information.
- Consider the purpose of the report.
- Consider your audience.

Presenting the report
- Be assertive.
- Speak clearly, calmly, and slowly.
- Avoid over-elaboration.
- Stick to your proposed task.
- Invite questions and comments.
- Be respectful of others.
- Stick to the time agreed.
- Make clear recommendations.
- Summarize main points at end.
- End with a clear take-home-message.

Patrick Callaghan, Professor of Mental Health Nursing, University of Nottingham & Nottinghamshire Healthcare NHS Trust

Further reading

www.askoxford.com

Writing and keeping records of care

Nurses have a professional responsibility to keep accurate records of the care they provide. The NMC acknowledge that record keeping is fundamental to nursing and provides guidelines for nurses on records and record keeping.

The importance of record keeping
- Helps to protect users' safety, health, and well-being.
- Promotes effective communication between different agencies involved in the care of users.
- Provides a written account of the care and treatment provided.
- Reflects the professional standing of nursing.
- Often the sign of a capable and safe nurse.
- May be used in legal proceedings and complaints.
- Needed for audit and risk management purposes.
- May be used for teaching and research purposes.

The content and style of records (NMC, 2002)
- Be factual, consistent, and precise.
- Write as soon as possible after an event has occurred.
- Write clearly and in such a manner that the text cannot be erased.
- Write the date, time, and sign all entries.
- Alterations should be dated, timed, and signed in a way that the original entry can still be read.
- Do not use abbreviations, jargon, meaningless phrases.
- Do not use irrelevant speculation.
- Do not use offensive subjective statements.
- Write entries, where possible with the involvement of users and their significant others.
- Write in way that can be understood by any reader.
- Write entries consecutively.
- Identify problems that have arisen and any action to rectify them.
- Provide clear evidence of the assessment, care planned, actions taken, information shared, and evaluation.

Access to, and storage of, records
Records held on users must be stored safely and securely and unauthorized persons will not normally be allowed access to these records. The Access to Health Records Act (1990) defines the rights of access of users to records held on them. The Data Protection Act (DPA) 1984 provides guidance on the safe and secure storage of information held about patients. Mental Health Nurses should not breach the DPA when holding records of users.

Helen Waldock, Health and Social Care Advisory Service

Further reading
Nursing and Midwifery Council. Guidelines for records and record keeping. NMC: London, 2002.

Discharge planning

Discharge planning is an essential component of mental health care, and one in which nurses play an active role. The Care Programme Approach (CPA) is the basis of caring for people with mental health problems; and planning for their discharge from hospital is central to its success. Effective discharge planning is especially important for users discharged on enhanced CPA.

The role of the mental health nurse
- Build discharge planning into care plans at the earliest opportunity.
- Contribute to CPA meetings that prepare the user for discharge.
- Work in partnership with the user and significant others in planning for discharge.
- Take a graded approach to discharge planning, e.g. accompanied visits to home and other facilities that the user will participate in after discharge.
- Liaise with other members of the care team and other agencies to ensure accurate and adequate exchange of information.
- Ensure the user has an adequate supply of medication post-discharge.
- Keep accurate written or electronic records of care provided.
- Ensure that users and significant others have details of who to contact in the event of problems after discharge.

The mental health nurse as care coordinator
- Oversee care planning and resource allocation.
- Keep in close contact with the user and significant others.
- Advise other members of the care team about changes in a user's circumstances that may warrant review.
- Update the user's care plan and crisis plan.

Requirements of the mental health nurse who is a care coordinator
- Competence in delivering mental health care.
- Knowledge of the service user and the family.
- Knowledge of community services and the role of other agencies.
- Coordination skills.
- Access to resources.

Patrick Callaghan Professor of Mental Health Nursing, University of Nottingham & Nottinghamshire Healthcare NHS Trust

Further reading

Department of Health. Effective Care Co-ordination in Mental Health Services: modernising the care programme approach. DoH: London, 2000.

Motivational interviewing

Motivational interviewing (MI) is a counselling method that is used in a range of health and social care settings and is designed to change health behaviour. MI is essentially client-centred, but it has a directive momentum, with the client presenting their own arguments for changing their behaviour. It is based on a collaborative alliance between the therapist and the client.[7] MI owes much to the work of Carl Rogers.[8]

Indications

MI is widely used in the treatment of problematic substance use, including smoking cessation; in treatment for lifestyle-related health problems, such as heart disease; and within the criminal justice system.

What does the therapist or counsellor do?

The focus of MI is not on the therapist's arguments for change, but rather on the client's own agenda. The client's own motivation for changing their behaviour is developed and worked on. By avoiding arguments, expressing empathy, supporting self-efficacy, and 'rolling with resistance,' an atmosphere of trust and acceptance is developed, where concerns about the behaviour can be explored.

It is important that the client is aware of the consequences of continuing the problematic behaviour. The therapist seeks to enable the client to highlight the discrepancy between what they want to achieve, and their current behaviour, highlighting how changing their behaviour will help them to achieve important goals.

The belief that change is possible is an important factor, and the instillation of hope is crucial.

Skills and techniques for MI
- Skilful reflective listening.
- Use of open ended and explanatory questions.
- Reflecting back information to the client as a statement, not a question.

Phases of motivational interviewing
- *Eliciting phase* – the therapist elicits self-motivating statements from the client.
- *Information phase* – the therapist actively seeks information from the client and may introduce a decision matrix.
- *Negotiation phase* – the therapist must value all decisions the client makes in this phase.

Eliciting self-motivational statements
A central part of the technique is listening for and reinforcing increases of positive expression in five key self-motivational areas:
- Self-esteem
- Concern about the behaviour
- Competence in other areas of the clients' life
- Knowledge of the problem and strategies to deal with it
- Desire for change.

Julie Attenborough City University, London

References

7 Miller, WR, Rollnick, S. *Motivational Interviewing: Preparing People for Change*. The Guilford Press: New York, 2002.

8 Rogers, CR. *Client-centred therapy*. Houghton-Mifflin: Boston, 1951.

Using rating scales

A rating scale is a device for measuring a person's reported state of mind or reported behaviour, performance, attitudes, intentions, abilities, personality, beliefs, cognitive functioning or style, preferences, and coping style. The term 'rating scale' is often used synonymously with test, inventory, questionnaire or measure.

The use of rating scales by mental health nurses

Rating scales can be useful in the following ways:

- They provide an assessment of users as a baseline, against which to measure the success of nursing interventions.
- They measure the behaviour of others.
- They report on aspects of people's state of mind or behaviour.
- During research as a tool to assess behaviour.
- During appraisal – as an assessment of performance.

Examples of rating scales used in mental health care

Rating scales are often used with interviews as part of a mental health assessment. Some commonly used rating scales in mental health are as follows:

- The Short Form-12 (SF-12) – a measure of general mental and physical health.
- The Health of the Nation Outcome Scale (HoNOS) – a measure of 12 categories of behaviour and mental state linked to mental health status.
- Brief Psychiatric Rating Scale (BPRS) – a measure of psychiatric symptoms.
- Edinburgh Post Natal Depression Scale (EPNDS) – a measure of depressive symptoms associated with childbirth.
- Beck Depression Inventory (BDI) – a measure of depressive symptoms.
- Side-Effects Checklist (SEC) – a measure of side-effects of drugs commonly used in psychiatry.
- Suicide Assessment and Management (SAM) – a measure of suicidal intent and previous self-harming behaviour.
- Social Functioning Scale (SFS) – A measure of day-to-day functioning that can be impaired by mental health problems.
- Carers' Assessment of Managing Index (CAMI) – A measure of stress and coping in people caring for people with mental health problems.
- Nurses' Observation Scale for In-patient Evaluation (NOSIE) – a measure of users' state of mind and behaviour in an in-patient mental health setting.
- Nurses' Evaluation Rating Scale (NERS) – A measure of users' behaviour in an inpatient setting that might indicate level of dependency.

Patrick Callaghan, Professor of Mental Health Nursing, University of Nottingham & Nottinghamshire Healthcare NHS Trust

Further reading

Andrews, G, Jenkins, R (eds.). *Management of Mental Disorders*, UK edn. WHO Collaborating Centre for Mental Health and Substance Misuse: Sydney, 1999.

Care of the survivor

Mental health services for survivors of violence should be part of a package of care that is founded on the needs of the individual survivor, rather than on a set of predetermined procedures. This is true whether the violence is intentional (e.g. partner abuse) or unintentional (e.g. a road traffic crash). The approach to care should be structured and contained within clear boundaries to provide psychological safety. There are many models on which care of survivors can be based; this chapter aims to provide a framework for practice.

Assessment

Assessment must be based on 'working with' rather than 'doing to' the survivor. The aim is always to avoid disempowering the client, and a non-judgemental attitude is essential from the outset. Respect for, and empathy with the client and the client's experiences are also key issues in avoiding disempowerment. Using an open and listening approach and avoiding an interrogative attitude will help the client to describe their personal experience.

Boundaries

Physical boundaries assist in containing the feelings and emotions of the client. For example;
- Timings – keep to previously agreed start and finish times.
- Location – this should be private, uninterrupted and comfortable, with the same room being used for later sessions.

Psychological boundaries are also important. For example;
- Keep all discussion with the client in the client-practitioner relationship.
- Keep discussion within the professional relationship focused on the event in question.

Personal boundaries should also be considered. For example;
- A client who has been assaulted may be very sensitive to an invasion of their personal space.

Outcome

The desired outcome is the long-term health of the client. It is therefore imperative that they are not re-victimized by whatever model of care is used. The practitioner must be aware of the possibility of the client being re-victimized by other processes such as cross examination in a court of law, or when asked by several different professionals to retell their story. A practitioner may be working with a client who is already re-victimized by the very processes that enabled them to survive. For example, in major incident management the focus may be on providing a standardized approach that could leave survivors unsupported in the first crucial hours after an event.

It is necessary to be gentle, and to allow space for the client to disclose in their own style and at their own pace.

Phillipa Sully & Malcolm Wandrag, City University, London

Crisis intervention

Many people with severe mental health problems, such as schizophrenia or bipolar affective disorder, enjoy long periods of relative well-being punctuated by episodes of acute illness. Acute episodes, or crises, can be triggered by a variety of factors, including environmental stressors.

Whilst people experience crises in individual ways, many will feel themselves overwhelmed and no longer able to cope. They may feel hopeless, have distressing thoughts or perceptual disturbances, and be unable to engage in everyday activities. People in crisis may also have thoughts of harming themselves or others, and be at risk of acting on these thoughts.

Interventions and services

Traditionally, mental health crises have been seen as problems to be managed within the hospital environment, often through the use of physical interventions including medication. However, alternatives to psychiatric hospital care have existed for many years. For example, in the UK, the Arbours Association has over three decades' experience in running a crisis centre for people in acute distress.[9] The development of user-led crisis services has also been supported by a leading charity, the Mental Health Foundation.[10]

In recent years, mainstream alternatives to hospital care have started to emerge, following the principle of providing services in the least restrictive environment. In the UK, new multidisciplinary crisis intervention and home treatment teams have appeared.[11] These aim to provide intensive, round-the-clock services, including therapeutic psychosocial interventions, rapid prescription and administration of medication, risk assessment and management, and help with practical activities. A systematic review of the effectiveness of services of this type found that:[12]

Home care crisis treatment, coupled with an ongoing home care package, is a viable and acceptable way of treating people with serious mental illnesses. If this approach is to be widely implemented, it would seem that more evaluative studies are needed.

Ben Hannigan, University of Cardiff

Good practice with people known to be vulnerable to crises includes the identification of early warning signs, and the construction of crisis management plans. These plans set out the actions to be taken in the event of acute episodes of ill-health. Both should be negotiated between practitioners, service users, and their carers.

References

9 www.arbourscentre.org.uk
10 www.mentalhealth.org.uk
11 Department of Health. The mental health policy implementation guide. DoH: London, 2001.
12 Joy, CB, Adams, CE, Rice, K. Crisis intervention for people with severe mental illnesses. In: *The Cochrane Database of Systematic Reviews*, vol 4. 2005. Oxford.

Social inclusion

People with mental health problems are among the most excluded in society. They have the lowest rate of employment of any disabled group; many have few friends and spend much of their time alone.

Social inclusion tackles this isolation and exclusion through the development of opportunities to engage in valued roles, relationships, and facilities, and support to access these opportunities.

Mental health nurses have a critical role in helping people move away from their identity as a stigmatized patient towards the role of recovering worker, student, parent, or friend, who can understand and manage their own mental health problems.

How mental health professionals can help promote social inclusion

Maintaining what people already have

People's roles and relationships are often lost through contact with mental health services. These need to be assessed from the start, so that friends, work, or college places are not lost, and a return to activities can be a planned and supported part of recovery.

Exploring new opportunities

Local listings, media outlets, and the Internet are all helpful in generating ideas about activities and facilities that might appeal to individuals, but it is also important to visit any facilities together with friends or family and find out what the expectations are before joining.

Helping individuals to access opportunities

It is helpful to plan and set targets if an individual is to meet their goals. Skills training might help develop confidence in particular situations. Adjustment of medication and ongoing support should be available at the level that is required.

Opportunities are more likely to be successful if the person is clear about what is expected, has an identified mentor or buddy, and has access to a mental health worker by phone. Time off for appointments, and appropriate adjustments to the physical environment to optimize the ability of the person to function should be negotiated from the start.

Dr Julie Repper, University of Sheffield

Increasing the capacity of communities
Target one particular organization and promote the inclusion of a person rather than an 'illness'. Explain the person's problems in everyday (not diagnostic) language, allow them to talk about their worries, and provide a contact point for advice. The person is usually their own best advocate – so involve them as much as possible.

Further reading

Department of Health. Mental Health and Social Exclusion. Social Exclusion Unit, Office of the deputy Prime Minister: London, 2004.
Repper, J, Perkins, R. *Social Inclusion and Recovery: a model for mental health practice.* Bailliere Tindall: London, 2004.

Electroconvulsive Therapy (ECT)

ECT is a procedure that involves a brief application of an electric current to the brain, through the scalp, inducing a seizure. It is typically used to treat a person who is experiencing severe depression or acute mania.

ECT remains the most controversial treatment for psychiatric illness, although it has been used since the 1940s and 1950s. Many of the risks and side-effects have been related to the misuse of equipment, incorrect administration and improperly trained staff. There is also a misconception that ECT is used as a 'quick fix' instead of long-term therapy or hospitalization. Unfavourable news reports and media coverage have added to the controversy surrounding this treatment. ECT is generally safe and among the most effective treatments available for intractable depression.

How ECT is done

The procedure is performed by an anaesthetist, a psychiatrist, and a qualified ECT nurse.

Before

General anaesthesia is used for this procedure, so the patient will be advised to not eat or drink before ECT. Patients will also be given a muscle relaxant, so that there will be no movement of the body during the procedure.

During

Electrodes are placed on the patient's scalp and a finely controlled electric current is applied, which causes a brief seizure in the brain. Because the muscles are relaxed, the seizure will usually be limited to slight movement of the hands and feet. Patients are carefully monitored during ECT treatment. When they wake up, minutes later, they do not remember the treatment or events surrounding the treatment, and may be confused.

After

Side-effects may be caused by the anaesthesia or by the ECT itself, or by both. Immediate side effects that may occur within the first few hours after a treatment include:
- Headaches
- Muscle aches or muscle soreness
- Nausea
- Confusion

Helen Waldock, Health and Social Care Advisory Service

- Hypotension, low blood pressure
- Tachycardia – a heart rate that is faster than normal, may accompany a bounding pulse.
- Allergic reaction to the anaesthesia
- Loss of memory for some events that occurred around the time of the treatment is common. This memory loss improves, but some patients have persisting gaps in memory for that time period. These will need to be monitored by the nurse.

Further reading

National Institute for Clinical Excellence. Guidance on the use of Electroconvulsive Therapy. NICE: London 2003.

Challenging behaviour

Challenging behaviour is a term used to describe behavioural distress. It is most often used by those caring for people with learning disabilities, or children and adolescents, but it is also used by those caring for people with mental health problems.

Definitions

Challenging behaviour is defined as:

> 'behaviour of such intensity, frequency or duration that the physical safety of the person or others is likely to be placed in serious jeopardy, or behaviour which is likely to seriously limit or deny access to, and use of, ordinary community facilities' (Emerson et al., 1987).

The Mental Health Foundation have expanded on this to include behaviour that is likely to

> 'impair an individual's personal development and family life and which represents a challenge to services, to families, and to the individual themselves, however caused.'[13]

Within mental health services, challenging behaviour is manifested by the following:
- Aggression
- Self injury
- Disruption and/or destruction of the environment
- Stereotyped or idiosyncratic behaviour.

Examples of these behaviours in people with mental health problems range from intimidating others, self harming behaviours such as cutting, and regressed behaviours such as refusing to self-care. Mental health professionals may label such behaviours as 'attention-seeking'; this is often an indication of staff frustration and possible power struggles.

Management of challenging behaviour

Managing challenging behaviour requires an understanding of the underlying motivation. This motivation can be divided into two broad categories; an inability to communicate frustration or a need in a more acceptable manner, or as a means of controlling their environment. Any strategy designed to manage challenging behaviour must consider that it may be reinforced by the response of others. Strategies for managing challenging behaviour involve setting limits non-punitively. Before setting these limits:
- Carers should state their expectations of the client in a positive, rather than a negative way.
- Explore the reasons for, and meaning of, the behaviour with the client, and consider alternatives.
- Inform the client which behaviours are, and are not, acceptable, and explain the consequences for behaving unacceptably.

Lynny Turner, City University, London

Once these issues have been clarified with the client, the consequences of unacceptable behaviour must occur. Firm, but not hostile, enforcement of limits is essential. Success requires that every member of the care team is consistent in their understanding of, and response to, the limits set. The care team does not assume responsibility for the client's behaviour, whether positive or negative. The client retains the right to choose how he or she behaves, as long as the consequences are clear.

Reference

13 Mental Health Foundation. MHF: www.mentalhealth.org.uk. Updates Vol 3 Issue 19, June, 2002.

Further reading

Emerson, E, Toogood, A, Mansell, J, *et al.* Challenging behaviour and community services: 1. Introduction and overview. *Mental Handicap* **15**, 166–9, 1987.

Occupational stress in the mental health workforce

Stress can be defined as

'a condition in which there is a marked perceived discrepancy between the demands on an individual and the individual's ability to respond, the consequences of which may be detrimental to future conditions essential for bio-psycho-social equilibrium and general well-being.'[14]

In the UK, an estimated half a million employees believe they are experiencing stress, anxiety and/or depression as a direct result of work.[15] Evans et al. in a national survey of stress levels amongst 237 mental health social workers, found substantial levels of stress and burnout, amounting to approximately double the levels reported for psychiatrists.[16]

Factors leading to this included feeling undervalued at work, excessive work demands, little control over decision-making, and an overall concern about the low status of the mental health social workers compared to other professional groups. Edwards et al. examined studies on burnout and stress for all members of the mental health multidisciplinary team, and 11 studies specifically on Community Mental Health Nurses. The evidence suggested that members of community mental health teams are experiencing increasing levels of stress and burnout.[17]

The major stress factors for community mental health nurses are:

- Job based stressors: increases in workload and administration, time management problems, inappropriate referrals, and violent and suicidal clients.
- Role based stressors: role conflict, responsibility and role change, lack of time for personal study.
- Stressors relating to organizational structure and climate such as NHS and legislative reforms.
- Stressors relating to relationships with others such as inadequate supervision and dysfunctional community mental health teams.

Professor Peter Ryan, Middlesex University

There is a growing body of evidence to suggest that mental health workers experience considerable stress in the course of carrying out their work. This stress and burnout not only affect the level of performance and the success of their interventions, but also job satisfaction and ultimately their own health.[18] Structural costs in terms of absenteeism, loss of productivity, and use of health service resources are inevitable consequences.

References

14 Rabin, S, Feldman, D, Kaplan, Z. Stress and Intervention Strategies in Mental Health Professionals. *British Journal of Medical Psychology* **72**: 159–69, 1999.
15 Mental Health Foundation. The Fundamental Facts. MHF: London, 1999.
16 Evans, S, Huxley, P, Gately, C, et al. Mental Health, Burnout and Job Satisfaction Among Mental Health Social workers in England and Wales. *British Journal of Psychiatry* **188**: 75–80, 2006.
17 Edwards, D, Burnard, P, Coyle, D, et al. Stress and burnout in community mental health nursing: a review of the literature. *Journal of Psychiatric and Mental Health Nursing* **7**: 7–14, 2000.
18 Carson, J, Cooper, C, Fagin, L, et al. Coping Skills in Mental Health Nursing: Do they make a Difference? *International Journal of Social Psychiatry* **42**(2): 102–11, 1996.

Working with homeless people with a mental health problem

Mental illness in homeless people may present in the form of schizophrenia, depression and other affective disorders, psychoses (including drug-induced psychosis), anxiety states, or personality disorder. Mental illness is the entry into homelessness for some people. Approximately 20 per cent of homeless people with mental ill-health are also diagnosed with substance dependence. Less than one third of homeless people with mental illness actually receive treatment.

Homelessness and extreme poverty are distant realities for many of us. Our brief encounters with homeless people reinforce prejudices and perceptions that influence our practice as health care professionals. Without prejudices we are better health care providers; it is therefore essential to understand both the circumstances that lead to homelessness, and the consequences of living on the street or in shelters.

Causes of homelessness

These can include:
- Lack of affordable housing or poverty.
- Substance misuse and lack of appropriate services.
- Mental illness.
- Domestic violence, abuse in the home.
- Relationship breakdown (partners and children).
- Prison release.
- Changes or cuts in public services.

Consequences of homelessness

These can include:
- Coronary heart disease – a major cause of death in the homeless (up to three times higher that the general population) due to smoking and substance abuse, nutritional inadequacies, and under-treated co-morbidities.
- Suicide – a higher than average possibility among the homeless.
- Respiratory complaints – very common in the inner-city population e.g. asthma or chronic lung disease due to the high prevalence of smoking. Compromised pulmonary status, coupled with the risks of homelessness, increases the probability of infection.
- HIV and AIDS – may result in job loss, with subsequent difficulty establishing eligibility for disability benefits, and the social stigma of the disease.
- Gastrointestinal conditions – those of concern include liver disease, and peptic ulcers due to the high rate of smoking.
- Family planning, pregnancy, and child-care issues – particularly for homeless women.
- Dermatological disorders – skin diseases such as psoriasis, eczema, and dermatitis can be neglected until they become disabling.
- Deterioration of existing mental health problems – and the development of other mental health problems.

Helen Waldock, Health and Social Care Advisory Service

Homelessness can be regarded as a continuum with rooflessness at one end and secure accommodation at the other. In between are degrees of fragile and insecure arrangements, such as a friend's floor or a night shelter; which leave people vulnerable to psychological stressors.

Working with the homeless requires:
- Accurate diagnosis – they may have complex presentations and histories.
- Recognition of co-morbidity.
- Awareness of social exclusion and contributing factors – not having an address means they are unable to register with a doctor.
- Active case management at an inter-agency level.
- Assertive community treatment programmes integrating mental health and social care.
- Street outreach programmes.
- Accurate risk assessment and risk management.

Further reading

Bhugra, D. Homelessness and mental health. Cambridge University Press: Cambridge, 1996.

Working with women with mental health problems

Introduction

Women are more likely than men to suffer from depression, eating disorders, and anxiety. Women often attribute their mental ill health to multiple demands (from family and work), overload (no time to rest) and isolation or lack of confidence. Women tend to focus not on personal culpability, but on the impact of the social situation (work and family, culture, religion, social class, marital status) in which they find themselves.

Women expect services that:
- Ensure safety.
- Promote empowerment and choice.
- Emphasize the underlying causes and context of women's distress.
- Value women's strengths, abilities, and potential for recovery.

Suggestions for gender sensitive practice

- Involve women in decisions about their treatment and recovery.
- Enable women to choose the sex of workers providing physical and mental health care.
- Provide women-only spaces within the physical environment of the service.
- Address issues of importance to women at various stages of their lives, e.g. menstruation, parenting, menopause, physical health, side-effects of medication (especially weight gain), sexual abuse, domestic violence, body image and sexuality.
- Provide practical help with housing and financial issues, education and employment, and flexibility around child care arrangements.
- Create opportunities for women to share with and learn from others who have had similar experiences.
- Provide women-only therapy groups, especially for issues such as domestic violence or sexual abuse.
- Advocate for women who are not able to voice their needs or stand up for themselves, e.g. in consultations where several different professionals are present.
- Collate and disseminate information about locally available resources and contacts for women.
- Acknowledge women's internal and external resources, such as personal coping strategies, strengths and social networks.
- Attempt to understand a woman's distress in the context of her life as a whole. For example, an unresolved history of physical, sexual, or emotional abuse may be impacting on their current mental health.
- Acknowledge that behaviours such as self-harm, disordered eating, or substance misuse may have meaning for the women concerned, and they may need help to understand and explore this.

Professor Sara Owen, University of Lincoln

Other considerations
- Planning pregnancy.
- The impact of pregnancy on medication concordance and mental well being.
- Post partum care for those with a known mental health problem.
- Child protection procedures.
- Care of the vulnerable adult.

Further reading
Barnes, M, Rogers, H. Women-Only and Women-Sensitive Mental Health Services: Expert Briefing Paper. NIMHE: Leeds, 2003.
Department of Health. Women's Mental Health: Into the Mainstream. DoH, London, 2002.
Both documents available at: www.nimhe.org.uk

Working with people with a perceptual disorder

A perceptual disorder is when a person's psychological experiences cause them severe distress or severe disability. These experiences are either additional to normal (positive symptoms, e.g. hallucinations) or detracting from normal experience (negative symptoms e.g. social withdrawal).

Relationship building

Basic principles of honesty and respect are the cornerstones of any work. Within this, the clinician must be honest in terms of what they can and cannot offer. They must appreciate that the user's experiences may seem bizarre or irrational to them, but that they are real to the user, who must always be treated with consideration.

Assessment

The aim of an assessment is to gain a shared understanding of both positive and negative symptoms. It is essential that this is carried out and recorded as a baseline for future progress to be measured against.

Example of assessments
- Brief Psychiatric Rating Scale (BPRS).
- Psychotic Symptom Rating Scales (PSYRATS).
- Positive and Negative Syndrome Scale (PANSS).

Intervention

Assessment should give the lead to intervention. Users may receive different combinations of the following, depending on the problem that causes them most distress, or is the most debilitating:

1. Psychiatric medication
Psychiatric medication is used to balance neurotransmitters thought to influence the user's experience e.g. perception. Users should be made aware of side-effects associated with any medication, and encouraged to monitor these for themselves.

2. Problem and symptom focused psychosocial interventions (PSI)
With PSI the user is offered a menu of interventions to distract their mind away from their symptoms (distraction) or to explore their symptoms and experiment with changing and controlling them (focusing).

3. Social skills training
Social skills training aims to increase the person's ability in social interactions. It utilizes role-play, practice, and homework in a safe environment.

4. Family interventions
These are aimed at assisting families to support the user by offering education and problem solving.

Geoff Brennan, Prospect Park Hospital, Tilehurst, Berkshire

Evaluation

Measuring the outcome of an intervention against the assessment baseline gives the evaluation of effectiveness. Other issues such as benefits, accommodation, and employment needs should be considered if these are identified issues for the client.

Further reading

Gamble, C, Brennan, G. *Working with Serious Mental Illness: A Manual for Clinical Practice*, 2nd edn. Bailliere Tindall: London, 2005.

Working with the client with a mood disorder

The term 'mood disorder' usually means depression and bipolar disorder. Biological, psychological, and social stressors increase a person's vulnerability to a mood disorder. Stressors are not always identified but include:

- Physical problems such as chronic pain or illness.
- Mood altering drugs and alcohol.
- Loss (e.g. role, health, youth).
- Unhappy life experiences leading to low self-esteem and poor coping.
- Acute personal crisis.
- Ongoing difficulties (e.g. relationships, school, work, money).

Extreme or very rapid changes in mood with a deteriorating quality of life, or presenting a risk to self or others, may require intervention.

Key points for intervention

The same range of treatments should be offered to adults of all ages. Ongoing monitoring is always required.

Mild depression

- Often self-limiting.
- Consider psychological treatments.

Moderate and severe depression, psychotic depression, and bipolar disorder

Consider:
- Medication.
- Psychological treatments.

Nursing role

General

- Be knowledgeable and competent in your role.
- Continually assess mood and risk.
- Establish a therapeutic alliance, with the client as an equal partner.
- Whenever possible, involve family and friends.
- Maintain professional boundaries.
- Provide accurate information in a clear and sensitive way.

Psychological factors

Risk of reduction in motivation, self-esteem, and confidence.
- Encourage self-management – through a better understanding of the impact of triggers, their prevention, and treatment.
- Anxiety management.
- Positive reinforcement.

Social factors

Risk of social isolation.
- Collaborate on structured goal setting to encourage social activity.

Professor Karina Lovell & Sarah Kendall, University of Manchester

Biological factors
Risk of self neglect.
- Health education – provide accurate information and encourage and support improvements in:
  - Sleep
  - Exercise
  - Diet
  - Fluid intake
  - Rest.
- Medication concordance – liaise with prescribers and provide accurate information about medication, including unwanted effects. Discourage other mood-altering substances.
- Encourage a low stimulus environment – this is especially important for clients with elevated mood. Take care with levels of lighting, noise, and activity.

Risk associated with working with the person with a mood disorder
Increased impulsive and high risk behaviour including self-harm and suicide attempts. Ongoing monitoring is necessary.
- Reduce access to potentially harmful substances and situations
- Devise a collaborative risk management plan including:
  - Close monitoring
  - Assessment of available resources
  - Risk reduction strategies
  - Communication with carers
  - Crisis plan.

Further reading
Newell, R, Gournay, K (eds.). *Mental Health Nursing-evidence based approach*. Churchill Livingstone: London, 2003.
National Institute for Clinical Excellence. Clinical Guideline 23; Depression, Management of depression in primary and secondary care. NICE: London, December 2004. www.nice.org.uk

Working with people with anxiety disorder

Fear is one of the universal basic emotions that is not learned and occurs across cultures. The fear/anxiety response is a basic survival response that helps an organism deal with threat or danger. Fear has been described as a 'usually unpleasant response to realistic danger', whereas anxiety is 'similar to fear but without the objective source of danger'. Anxiety symptoms and disorders are prevalent and co-exist within a range of mental health disorders.

Anxiety symptoms
Physiological symptoms
- *Cardiovascular* – palpitations, heart racing
- *Respiratory* – rapid breathing, shortness of breath
- *Neuromuscular* – tremors, fidgeting
- *Gastrointestinal* – abdominal discomfort, nausea
- *Skin* – face flushed or pale.

Behavioural symptoms
- Inhibition
- Flight or avoidance
- Restlessness
- Impaired coordination.

Cognitive symptoms
- Sensory-perceptual – hazy or foggy mind, feelings of unreality
- Thinking difficulties – confusion, difficulty concentrating
- Conceptual – fear of losing control or going mad.

Assessment and treatment questionnaires
- Problem assessment
- Mental state examination
- Full history assessment
- The fear questionnaire
- The Beck anxiety and depression inventory.

Main interventions
The two main interventions for anxiety disorders are exposure and cognitive behaviour therapy. There is a limited evidence base for the effectiveness of relaxation therapies in relieving anxiety.

Exposure
Exposure can be defined as 'facing something that causes fear and has been avoided.' 'In-vivo' exposure refers to exposure in real life, where the client is actually in the presence of the feared stimulus or situation. 'Imaginal' exposure is where the client is asked to produce an image or mental description of their most feared situation.

Professor Paul Rogers, University of Glamorgan

When planning an exposure programme, careful assessment will reveal the range of internal and external stimuli that will reliably elicit an anxiety response. It is important that the client understands what is involved and the reasons for treatment.

Cognitive behaviour therapy (CBT)

The initial assessment and focus of CBT is on the person's automatic thoughts that reflect their ongoing appraisal of events in their lives. This is aided by the use of an assessment diary – where the person monitors emotional changes thus allowing identification of the negative thoughts that preceded them. Clark has identified the active ingredients of cognitive therapy for anxiety disorders as: education, verbal discussion techniques, imagery modification, attentional manipulation, exposure to feared stimuli, manipulation of safety behaviours and other behavioural experiments.[19]

Reference

19 Clark, DA. Anxiety disorders: why they persist and how to treat them. *Behaviour Research* and *Therapy* **37**: S5–S27, 1999.

Further reading

Hawton, K, Salkovkis, P, Kirk, J et al. (eds.). *Cognitive Behaviour Therapy for Psychiatric Problems: A Practical Guide*. Oxford University Press: Oxford, 1989.

Marks, IM. *Fears, Phobias and Rituals: panic, anxiety and their disorders*. Oxford University Press: Oxford, 1987.

Working with a person with anorexia nervosa

There are five categories of eating disorder, identified by the Diagnostic and Statistical Manual of Mental Disorders (DSM IV). This chapter focuses on anorexia nervosa.

Diagnostic criteria

The diagnostic criteria for anorexia nervosa are:
- Body weight of at least 15 below normal for age, height, and body frame.
- Self-induced weight loss.
- Perception of being too fat.
- Body image disturbance (eg feeling fat when emaciated).
- Absence of three consecutive menstrual cycles.
- Denial of seriousness of low body weight.

Epidemiology

The overall prevalence in the general population is probably less than 1%. Females account for between 70 and 95% of all cases, and males 5–15%. Clinical samples show the `typical' presentation is a 15–25 year old female, of upper socioeconomic status. Community samples show a more equitable distribution across different socio-economic groups.

Assessment

An assessment interview establishes the needs of the person, and agrees a therapeutic contract, if required. A brief assessment might involve determining how the client views the issue, assessing for any specific or general psychopathology, social circumstances/functioning, and physical health status. Psychometric measures used in the assessment process include: The Eating Attitudes Test (EAT), Body Shape Questionnaire (BSQ), and Setting Conditions for Anorexia Nervosa Scale (SCANS).

NICE Guidelines (clinical guideline 9) on the treatment and management of anorexia nervosa

Recommendations from NICE include:
- Assessment and management should occur in primary care.
- Helpful psychological interventions are: Cognitive Analytic Therapy, CBT, and Interpersonal Psychotherapy.
- Physical management should include managing weight gain, nutritional re-stabilization, and managing risk.

Mental health nursing care of people with anorexia nervosa

- Assess readiness to change. (☐ Motivational interviewing.)
- Exploration of the person's view.
- Probe for signs and symptoms that cause concern to the person and their significant others.
- Identify the pros and cons for the person of anorexia nervosa.
- Provide an alternative for unhealthy behaviours.

Patrick Callaghan, Professor of Mental Health Nursing, University of Nottingham & Nottinghamshire Healthcare NHS Trust

Recognizing the onset of anorexia nervosa

The following *may* indicate the onset of a potential eating disorder:

- Sudden changes in eating behaviour or pattern.
- Over-involved interest in body shape and image.
- Excessive dieting behaviour, especially when weight is normal.
- Marked changes in mood, loss of menarche or failure to establish menarche.
- Severe weight loss.
- Emaciated appearance.

Possible triggers for anorexia nervosa

- Taunts about body shape and weight.
- Acne and taunts about this.
- Family conflict.
- Educational or work pressures to succeed.
- Other illnesses e.g. thyroid problems.
- Growing up in a 'dieting culture'.
- Relationship difficulties.
- Reactions to loss.

Prognosis

About 54% of people with anorexia nervosa recover. The illness has a mortality rate of 10–15%. Most of these die of physical complications, and around 33% commit suicide. Predictors of an unfavourable outcome are purging, physical symptoms, advanced age at presentation, and high social status.

Further reading

National Institute of Clinical Excellence. Core interventions in the treatment and management of anorexia nervosa, bulimia nervosa and related eating disorders, Clinical Guideline 9. NICE: London, 2004.

Treasure, J, Carolan, A, Todd, G. The Person with an Eating Disorder. In: I Norman, I Ryrie (eds.) *The Art and Science of Mental Health Nursing: A Textbook of Principles and Practice.* Open University Press: Buckingham, 2004: pp. 457–80.

Working with a person with bulimia nervosa

The Diagnostic and Statistical Manual of Mental Disorders (DSM IV) published by the American Psychiatric Association, identifies five categories of eating disorders. These are anorexia nervosa, bulimia nervosa, pica rumination disorder of infancy, feeding disorder of infancy or early childhood, and unspecified eating disorder. This chapter focuses on bulimia nervosa.

Diagnostic criteria

The diagnostic criteria for bulimia nervosa are:
- Episodes of compulsive binge eating.
- Lack of control over eating binges.
- Use of extreme methods for controlling weight e.g. self-induced vomiting, laxative abuse, diuretic abuse, restrictive dieting, or vigorous exercise.
- At least two binge eating episodes per week for at least three months.
- Obsessive concern with body shape, body weight, and body size.
- The behaviour does not occur exclusively during episodes of anorexia nervosa.

Epidemiology

Estimates of the overall prevalence of bulimia nervosa suggest 1.3% for females and 0.1% for males. Some college studies report rates of between 12.5% and 18.6%.

Assessment

An assessment interview is necessary to establish the needs of the client and agree a therapeutic contract, if required. A brief assessment might involve determining how the client views the issue, assessing for any specific or general psychopathology, social circumstances, social functioning and physical health status. Psychometric measures used in the assessment process include The Eating Attitudes Test (EAT) and the Body Shape Questionnaire (BSQ).

NICE Guidelines on the management and treatment of bulimia nervosa

Recommendations from NICE include:
- Helpful psychological interventions are: CBT, self-help, or Interpersonal Psychotherapy as an alternative to CBT.
- Helpful pharmacological interventions are: antidepressants such as SSRIs.
- Management of physical aspects should include: assessment of fluid and electrolyte balance; plus an oral supplement if there are imbalanced fluids and electrolytes.

Patrick Callaghan, Professor of Mental Health Nursing, University of Nottingham & Nottinghamshire Healthcare NHS Trust

Mental health nursing care of person with bulimia nervosa

- Assess readiness to change (📖 Motivational interviewing).
- Exploration of the person's illness perception.
- Probe for signs and symptoms that cause concern to the person and significant others.
- Identify the pros and cons of bulimia nervosa.
- Provide an alternative for unhealthy behaviours.

Recognizing the onset of bulimia nervosa

The following *may* indicate the onset of a potential eating disorder:

- Sudden changes in eating behaviour or pattern.
- Over-involved interest in body shape and image.
- Excessive dieting behaviour especially when weight is normal.
- Marked changes in mood, loss of menarche or failure to establish menarche.
- Severe weight loss.
- Emaciated appearance.
- Excessive teeth brushing and prolonged visits to the toilet after every meal.

Many people with bulimia experience the decay of dental enamel caused by hydrocloric acid passing through the mouth during episodes of vomiting. Frequent dental visits are often necessary.

Factors which may trigger bulimia nervosa

- Taunts about body shape and weight.
- Taunts about appearance, e.g. acne.
- Family, educational, or work pressures to succeed.
- Other problems, e.g.
  - growing up in a 'dieting culture'.
  - relationship difficulties.
  - reactions to loss.

Prognosis

The prognosis for bulimia nervosa is good on the whole. Predictors of an unfavourable outcome are significant loss of self-esteem or severe personality disorder.

Further reading

National Institute of Clinical Excellence. Core interventions in the treatment and management of anorexia nervosa, bulimia nervosa and related eating disorders, Clinical Guideline 9. NICE: London, 2004.

Treasure, J, Carolan, A, Todd, G. The Person with an Eating Disorder. In: I Norman, I Ryrie (eds.) *The Art and Science of Mental Health Nursing: A Textbook of Principles and Practice.* Open University Press: Buckingham, 2004: pp. 457–80.

Working with the person with substance misuse problems

Substance misuse is a major public health problem and is associated with a number of common mental health problems. Persistent or recurrent problems with substance misuse are defined as either:

- Harmful use – substance use which causes actual damage to physical or mental health for at least one month, or repeatedly; or
- Dependence syndrome – a group of behavioural, physiological, and cognitive symptoms characterized by: compulsion to use, impaired control of intake, withdrawal states, tolerance, and continued use, despite a subjective awareness of adverse consequences.[20]

The use of lay terms in clinical settings (such as drug addict, alcoholic, or drug abuse) can further stigmatize people with substance misuse problems, encourages non-disclosure and should therefore be avoided.

The assessment process

A comprehensive assessment of substance misuse history, current problems, and physical and psychiatric co-morbidity are essential in planning effective care and support for service users, and should include the following basic elements:

- A full physical examination.
- Assessment of current substance use – use during the past month.
- Primary or other drug use – volume and frequency, route of administration, any prescribed drugs?
- A urine screen – to confirm history, especially where substitute prescribing is being considered.
- Past substance use history – including age of first use (and substances used), pattern, and progression of use.
- Social and personal circumstances – relationships, social and support network, children, housing status, employment, use of leisure time, interests.
- Reasons for and function of substance use.
- Subjective awareness of the problem.
- Periods of coerced or voluntary abstinence.
- Current contact with substance misuse service.
- Current and past treatment episodes – length and type of treatment (e.g. residential, rehabilitation, community detoxification). What worked? What didn't work and why?
- Assessment of risk – current or past injecting use? HIV and hepatitis status, home circumstances, safety, and use.
- Physical and mental health – acute or long-term medical issues, including any history of overdose. Current or previous mental health service contact.

Peter Phillips, City University, London

- Association between use and psychiatric symptoms (e.g. exacerbation, self-medication, relapses).
- Legal and forensic issues – current or previous contact with criminal justice system, including probation, funding of substance use, outstanding charges, type of offences (acquisitive or violent).

References

20 World Health Organization. Pocket Guide to the ICD-10 *Classification of Mental and Behavioural Disorders*. Churchill Livingstone: Edinburgh: 1994.

Principles of working with service users with substance misuse problems

Substance misuse is a common and increasing social phenomenon. It is often seen in mental health services, both as a 'primary' problem, and as a co-morbidity with mental illness. Substance misuse problems can include the misuse of alcohol, illicit substances e.g. prescribed medicines.

A positive therapeutic attitude in health workers is strongly associated with better clinical outcomes in people with substance misuse problems.

Approaches and interventions

Clinical interventions should be based on a comprehensive assessment of substance use history and current use (📖 Chapter 1, Introduction).

Interventions and service contact should match the severity of the illness or problem, and the stage of change that the person is at (see below). There are a number of interventions aimed at increasing motivation to change, and these include: increasing awareness of the need to change, increasing concern about current use, and use as a frustration of goals. Other interventions that are useful in working with substance users include: motivational interviewing and relapse prevention methods, including the use of matrices (📖 Motivational interviewing).

The stages of change

This is also known as the cycle of change[21] and includes: pre-contemplation, contemplation, decision, active change, maintenance, and relapse.

Most users are at least ambivalent about their substance use, and this ambivalence, linked with other adverse events (such as relapses or pre-cipitation of illness) can be used to help the service user move further in the cycle of change.

Harm reduction

Therapeutic work with service users with substance misuse problems should initially be focused on reducing substance related harms for the person, their family, friends and community. Subsequently, it should look at the reduction of actual substance use.

It is now widely recognized that the so-called 'harm reduction' approach to managing substance misuse problems is pragmatic, user-focused, and meets users 'as they are' with no hard and fast rules. It acknowledges the social context of much substance misuse.

Peter Phillips, City University, London

Harm reduction approaches should be seen on a continuum with abstinence at one end, and 'safer' use at the other. It may use a plethora of clinical tools including substitute prescribing, needle and syringe exchange programmes (where appropriate), drug education, and user involvement.

Reference

21 Prochaska, JO, Di-Clemente, CC. Towards a comprehensive model of change. In: WR Miller, N Heather (eds.) *Treating Addictive Behaviours: process of change*. Plenum Press: New York, 1982.

Further reading

Carey, K. Substance Use Reduction in the Context of Outpatient Psychiatric Treatment: A Collaborative, Motivational, Harm Reduction Approach. *Community Mental Health Journal* **3**(32): 291–306, 1996.

Assessing children and adolescents

Growing up takes time – perhaps as much as 20 to 25 years. Even then, many people consider they still have some way to go. Within this time span, difficulties will be encountered, problems will arise and conflicts will develop.

Mental health nurses may be asked to assess a child or adolescent who is having difficulty dealing with life's problems, but who will find resolutions eventually, without formal or professional interventions.

The Common Assessment Framework (DfSS 2004) offers an integrated approach to assessment and intervention. Local services should develop best collaborative practices for children and their families.

Child-centred focus

As they prepare to undertake an assessment, it is important for the professional to remind themselves that the child or adolescent they see is a unique individual, with his or her own individual capacities, strengths, and resilience. An assessment should seek to elicit these aspects as much as any risk factors, difficulty and/or signs and symptoms of underlying disturbance.

Issues to consider in the assessment process

Concerns

- Who has the concerns – the child, parent, teacher, or health professional?
- What are they concerned about – behaviour, relationships, school work?
- How does it manifest in the child or adolescent – the degree to which it interferes with day-to-day life?

Context

Assessment is undertaken with the following factors in mind:

- The child's developmental stage.
- The child's social and cultural context.
- Life events experienced by the child.

Global Assessment

Assessment is a systematic process of eliciting information about a child or adolescent that allows the professional to decide on an effective and appropriate level of intervention.

A holistic assessment framework (see Fig. 2.1) allows the professional to work systematically with the child and the family.

Factors specific to the child or adolescent

Psychological

- Behavioural issues.
- Development and meeting milestones.
- Attainment, coordination, selfcontrol.

Physical

- General health.
- Developmental norms – height, weight, puberty.

Who to involve in the assessment

You will need to discuss this with the child or adolescent, their parent(s) and siblings. With agreement, you may want to talk to staff from any agency or service involved. Decide who you will need information from and check that the child/adolescent/family are clear about this.

Jenny Cobb, City University, London

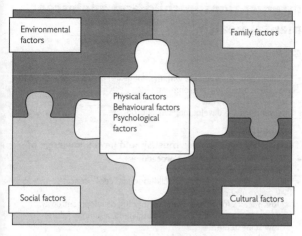

Fig. 2.1 Holistic assessment framework (J Cobb)

Factors that impact on the child or adolescent's experiences and relationships

Environmental
- Housing
- Local Service provision – schools, recreation and leisure
- Community facilities

Family
- Parenting styles – capacity to provide basic care
- Emotional availability – warmth, consistency
- Provide appropriate boundaries and guidance
- Siblings

Social
- Extended family groups
- Friendships
- Family history
- Employment and financial realities

Cultural
- Beliefs, religious or spiritual practices
- Peer group ethos
- Values and expectations

Assessment focus

Have you sufficient information to understand the child or adolescent's current position and to identify their needs? Can this information help clarify the factors that have triggered concern
- *Antecedents* – what was happening prior to the behaviour?
- *Precipitants* – what triggered the behaviour?
- *Perpetuators* – what maintains the behaviour?
- *Prognosis* – what are the chances of recovery?

Interventions in child and adolescent mental health

Core principles

It is important that:
- Children and young people with mental health problems are cared for in a safe and trusting environment.
- Care is family-centred.
- Interventions are developmentally appropriate.

Core knowledge

The mental health nurse must/should have knowledge of
- Child protection policies and procedures.
- Child development.
- Mental-ill health presenting in childhood and adolescence.
- Risk and resilience factors:
  - *Risk factors for a child:* genetics, low IQ, development delay, communication difficulties, physical illness, academic failure, low self-esteem.
  - *Resilience factors for a child:* self esteem, autonomy, sociability.
  - *Risk factors for a family:* parental conflict, family breakdown, inconsistent discipline, rejection, abuse, failing to meet development needs, parental psychiatric illness, parental criminality, death, or loss.
  - *Resilience factors for a family:* family compassion, warmth, no discord, good support.
- Interventions (see below).
- Family systems theories.

Core skills

The mental health nurse must/should have the following skills:
- Listening and attending.
- Communication and social skills.
- Observations of social interaction, play, mood, behaviour, sleep and diet.
- Formulating a care plan.
- Managing care (see below).

Care planning

When planning or managing care, the mental health nurse should:
- Remember that families are often involved with other services – consider these when planning care.
- Work in partnership with the child and family.
- Consider risk – be clear about how to keep children safe.
- What does the child and the family want to achieve? What are their goals and objectives?
- Negotiate child-centred interventions that are sensitive to difference, ethnicity and culture.
- Consider equipment – drawing paper, painting, human figures, animal figures and toys to facilitate communication.

Mariya Limerick, University of Nottingham

Interventions

These are interventions that may help children and adolescents:

- Counselling.
- Behavioural interventions – based on social learning theories, these help children and families to change their behaviour.
- Cognitive behavioural interventions – helps children understand how their thoughts and feelings affect their behaviour.
- Motivational interviewing – a communication technique to promote decision making and behaviour change.
- Solution-focused therapy – helps children work towards their own goals.
- Family therapy – looks at the family as an interconnected system of relationships. Skilled questioning and reflections help families discover ways to change. Example question, 'How do you think Eric feels when you shout at him?'
- Parent training – is based on social learning theories. It is structured, delivered on a sessional basis and helps improve parenting practices.
- Child psychotherapy – helps children and young people come to terms with complex emotional and relationship problems.
- Individual play therapy – helps children recover through communication and play.
- Creative therapies e.g. drama, art. and music – help children and young people express themselves and discover ways to change.
- Group therapy – provides support and an environment for change.
- Pharmacology – the most common medications are Ritalin (Methylphenidate) for ADHD (attention deficit hyperactivity disorder). Other drugs are used to treat psychosis and mood disorders.
- Intensive care – inpatient and day care facilities are suitable for more serious and persistent mental health problems.
- Multi-systemic therapy – wider systems are managed to ensure the young person receives a consistent package of care. Can be helpful with severe conduct disorder where education, youth justice, social services, and others are involved.

Further reading

Department of Health. National Service Framework for Children, Young people and Maternity Services. DoH: London, 2004.
DfES. Every Child Matters: Change for Children. DfES: London, 2004.
http://www.everychildmatters.gov.uk/key-documents/

Working with the person with personality disorder (PD)

Personality disorder is functional impairment or psychological distress resulting from inflexible and maladaptive personality traits. The person commonly presents with problems in thinking styles, emotional regulation, and impulse control, and has particular difficulties in relating to other people. These problems are long-standing and pervasive across a variety of situations.

The main types of PD are described in the two major diagnostic classification systems, the DSM-IV and ICD-10 (see table opposite). The three clusters have been derived from empirical work and are represented in terms of: A – odd eccentric behaviours; B – dramatic flamboyant and impulsive behaviour; and C – anxious and fearful behaviour.

It is important to understand that each different personality disorder consists of a varied collection of impairments, and therefore different presenting problems and issues. It is rare for someone to present with one personality disorder; co-morbidity is common.

People with cluster C anxiety based problems most often present in primary care settings, while those in cluster B tend to present to mental health services. Those in group B have often been associated with antisocial behaviour and deliberate self-harm, leading to problems of stigmatization and social exclusion from services.[22]

A minority of people with a personality disorder get the treatment they need in a forensic setting, after coming into contact with the police and the courts. This has led to many people with personality disorders being further stigmatized as representing a danger to society. Those people with antisocial PD in the forensic system tend to be the individuals who pose the greatest risk to others, whereas most people with PD are more at risk of harming themselves than other people.

Key issues in working with people with PD

Working with an individual with a personality disorder is challenging for nurses, as many of the problematic behaviours manifest in the person's interactions and relationships.

The following are important when working with people with PD:
- Supervision
- Effective team work
- Emotional support
- Knowledge and empathy for the traumatic and distressing histories that are common in this group.

Evidence-based interventions
- Cognitive behaviour therapy
- Cognitive analytic therapy
- Dialectic behaviour therapy
- Psychodynamic group therapy.

Dr Neil Gordon, Nottinghamshire Healthcare NHS Trust

Classifications of Personality Disorders

DSM IV	ICD-10
Cluster A	
Paranoid	Paranoid
Schizoid	Schizoid
Schizotypal	
Cluster B	
Antisocial	Dissocial
	Emotionally unstable
	a)Impulsive type
Borderline	b) Borderline type
Histrionic	Histrionic
Narcissistic	
Cluster C	
Avoidant	Anxious
Dependent	Dependent
Obsessive compulsive	Anankastic

Reference

22 NIMHE. No longer a diagnosis of exclusion. DoH: London, 2003.

Further reading

Bateman, A, Fonagy, P. The effectiveness of partial hospitalization in the treatment of borderline personality disorder – a randomized controlled trial. *American Journal of Psychiatry* **156**: 1563–9, 1999.

Livesley, J (ed.). *Handbook of personality disorders: Theory research and treatment.* The Guilford Press: New York, 2001.

Working with the person who uses forensic services

Forensic mental health services specialize in the assessment and treatment of people with mental health problems who are undergoing legal or court proceedings, or who have offended. People with mental health problems, who have never been involved with the criminal justice system, might also be treated in forensic psychiatric services, if they cannot be safely managed elsewhere.

Mental health nurses provide forensic interventions in healthcare and penal settings, including secure hospitals, the courts, prisons, and young offenders' institutions. The level of risk posed by an individual will dictate the level of security within which they are cared for. The range is from community services and low or medium secure hospitals to high secure hospitals with dangerous and severe personality disorder (DSPD) units. Most patients in these settings are detained under the Mental Health Act 1983.

Key skills in forensic nursing
- Psychological assessment
- Interpersonal and engagement skills
- Inter-agency working
- Risk assessment and management.

The offence for which a client is either charged or convicted is central to forensic nursing in any environment. Offences vary greatly, from the petty to the severe. The nurse's focus is working with the mental health issues that led to the offending behaviour.

Nurses need knowledge of therapeutic interventions, so they can rehabilitate clients with severe and enduring mental illnesses and personality related difficulties. They also need well developed support and supervison systems to help them process the emotional impact of this work.

CBT based psychotherapeutic approaches have been shown to be the most effective intervention for modifying some forms of difficult behaviour, as displayed by people presenting to forensic services. These treatments require time and special expertise, and are usually delivered by specialist multidisciplinary treatment teams.

Patrick Callaghan. Professor of Mental Health Nursing, University of Nottingham & Nottinghamshire Healthcare NHS Trust

People with mental health problems who have offended are often socially deprived and psychologically needy individuals who do not fit neatly into either the health or the penal system.[23] As a consequence, there is an increasing focus on developing hybrid services, combining the containment skills of the penal system with the therapeutic inputs of the health service. Nurses are key players in these developments, as the specialist nature of forensic practice is now being recognized and developed.

Reference

23 Webb, D, Harris, R. *Mentally disordered offenders: managing people nobody owns*. Routledge: London, 1999.

Further reading

Bowers, L. *Dangerous and Severe Personality Disorder: Reactions and Role of the Psychiatric Team.* Routledge: London, 2002.

Kettles, A, Woods, P, Collins, M. *Therapeutic Interventions for Forensic Mental Health Nurses.* Jessica Kingsley, London: 2001.

Working with the person who is suicidal and self-harms

People with mental health problems are at a greater risk of harming themselves than others. The rates of self-harm have continued to rise since the 1980s; and self-harming behaviour is a particular risk factor for suicide. About one quarter of all people who successfully commit suicide have attended hospital following an act of self-harm in the previous twelve months.[24]

Self-harming behaviour is commonly known as 'deliberate self-harm' or (DSH). DSH involves intentional self-poisoning or self-injury, irrespective of the apparent purpose of the act.[25] The two most common types of DSH are self-poisoning, such as an overdose, or cutting.

Who is at risk?

Men are three times more likely to commit suicide than women, although self-harm is more common among females, especially young women under the age of 25. The incidence of suicide increases with age, although there has been a recent increase in suicide among young adult men under 45. Suicide and self-harm are more common in white people than in other racial or ethnic groups. Social factors such as living alone, being homeless and unemployed are additional risk factors.[26]

Engagement and assessment

Self-harming patients most commonly access the health service through A&E departments, although this will depend on the nature and severity of harm caused. Successfully engaging with self-harming patients is challenging for healthcare professionals, as such behaviours can be difficult to comprehend and may challenge some of our most fundamental values and beliefs.

People who self-harm have complex needs, they may have problems in their lives and feel hopeless. Any risk assessment needs to address a number of different factors and to be part of a comprehensive package of care.

Therapeutic interventions

There are a number of strategies that can be employed to reduce self-harm or its repetition. The choice of therapeutic intervention should be based on the results of a comprehensive psychosocial assessment. DSH may be related to a person's depressed mental state, for example.

Dr Julia Jones, City University, London

Self-harming behaviour may not simply be attributed to a mental illness, but may also arise from social problems such as unemployment, debt or problems with personal relationships.

Existing research evidence suggests three useful interventions: problem solving therapy; the use of crisis cards; and dialectical behaviour therapy.

References

24 NHS Centre for Reviews and Dissemination. Deliberate Self Harm. *Effective Health Care* **4**(6): 1–12.
25 Hawton, K, Catalan, J. *Attempted Suicide: A Practical Guide to its Nature and Management.* Oxford University Press: Oxford, 1987.
26 Appleby L, *Five-Year report of the National Confidential Inquiry into Suicide and Homicide by People with Mental Illness*, DoH: London, 2001.

Interventions

Cognitive Behavioural Therapy (CBT)

Cognitive behavioural therapy (CBT) is a short-term problem-focused psychological intervention. It can be used to treat a number of psychiatric problems, including depression and anxiety. More recently, CBT has been used to reduce distress and improve functioning in more complex disorders, such as psychosis.

The cognitive behavioural model

The underlying theoretical rationale is that how we see the world and how we feel is influenced by our thoughts. We all have typical or automatic patterns of thinking that enable us to make quick evaluations of situations. In some people, there is a bias towards a particular type of thinking, such as negative thinking in depression.

Principles of cognitive behavioural approaches

Collaboration

The therapist structures the interview, but the patient identifies the problems that concern them. An inductive (or Socratic) style of questioning is used to help patients identify and explore their experience.

Setting goals and measuring outcome

Specific goals for treatments are identified. A range of tools are used to monitor outcomes such as questionnaires, diaries and worksheets.

Self-help

Patients are actively involved in monitoring their mood and their thinking. They learn how to apply the techniques, such as rating their own mood, and thereby modify their own thinking. The therapist will often set 'homework' so that the patient can continue the modification outside of the therapy session.

Assessment

This focuses on the problems the person faces in the present, in relation to the following areas:
- Life situation, relationships, and practical problems.
- Altered thinking.
- Altered emotions.
- Altered physical feelings or symptoms.
- Altered behaviour or activity levels.

Interventions

Cognitive interventions include identifying the thoughts that impacted on mood changing in a specific situation. A diary is used to record information, and over time, typical thinking patterns will start to emerge. Unhelpful thinking patterns are modified by techniques such as examining the evidence for the thoughts, and identifying the underlying beliefs.

Avoidance of particular activities and situations is a key feature of many problems, including anxiety and depression, and this contributes to

Madeline O'Carroll, City University, London

unhelpful thinking patterns. It can be addressed by structured or graded activities.

How effective is CBT?

- CBT is superior to befriending, especially in the long-term in people with persistent symptoms of schizophrenia, which are resistant to medication.
- CBT plus standard care is better than standard care alone in reducing relapse rates in people living with schizophrenia.
- CBT significantly benefits physical functioning in adult outpatients with chronic fatigue syndrome (CFS) when compared with relaxation or medical management.
- CBT is beneficial for anxiety disorders, phobias, OCD, chronic pain, PTSD, depression, and chronic fatigue.

Further reading

Grant, A, Mills, J, Mulhern, R, et al. Cognitive Behavioural Therapy in Mental Health Care. Sage Publications: London, 2004.

Jones, C, Cormac, I, Mota, J, et al. Cognitive behaviour therapy for schizophrenia (Cochrane Review). In: The Cochrane Library, issue 2. Update Software: Oxford, 2000.

Family Therapy

Family therapy (or **family systems therapy**) is a branch of psychotherapy that treats family problems. Family therapists consider the family as a system of interacting members; as such, the problems in the family are seen to arise as an emergent property of the interactions in the system, rather than being ascribed exclusively to the 'faults' or psychological problems of individual members.

A **family** is a domestic group of people, or a number of domestic groups, typically affiliated by birth or marriage, or by comparable legal relationships including domestic partnership, adoption, or surname. Although many people have understood familial relationships in terms of 'blood,' it has been argued that the notion of 'blood' must be understood metaphorically, and in that in many societies family is understood through other concepts rather than 'blood.' This is especially true when considering the cultural or sexual preference considerations of an individual.

A family therapist usually sees several members of the family at the same time in therapy sessions. This setting has the advantage of making differences between the ways different family members perceive mutual relations as well as interaction patterns in the session apparent both for the therapist and the family. These patterns frequently mirror habitual interaction patterns at home, even though the therapist is now incorporated into the family system. Therapy interventions usually focus on these patterns of interaction rather than analysing subconscious impulses or early childhood traumas of individuals as a Freudian therapist would do.

Depending on circumstances, the therapist may then point out to the family these interaction patterns that the family might have not noticed; or suggest to individuals a different way of responding to other family members. These changes in the way of responding may then trigger repercussions in the whole system, sometimes leading to a more satisfactory system state.

Family work and mental illness

Expressed emotion: is a measure of how well relatives of a mentally ill patient express their attitude towards them while they are not present. Expressed emotion is a huge factor during the recovery process of those diagnosed with psychological illnesses. The three attitudes pertaining to expressed emotion are known as hostile, critical, and emotional over-involvement.

Criticalness: the combination of hostile and emotional over-involvement, where the family is in denial about any mental health issue and associated behavioral issues.

Emotional over-involvement: family members blame themselves instead of the patient for everything, they feel everything is their fault and they feel sorry for the person who is ill.

Helen Waldock, Health and Social Care Advisory Service

Hostility: the family member puts blame on the patient because of their illness, believing them to be foolish and selfish, and holding them accountable for any negative action that arises.

Those who have expressed high emotion tend to be more negative than the ones who are low. The attitudes of the relatives determine the direction of the illness after treatment. The relatives influence the outcome of the disorder through negative comments and nonverbal actions. These particular interactions between family members who are dealing with a patient with a psychological disorder are stressful for the recovering patient. The pressure from the family for the patient to recover and to end certain behaviours can cause the person a relapse in their illness.

Further reading

Piercy, FP. Family Therapy Source Book. Guilford Publishing: 1996.
Rasheed, JM, Keung, HM. Family Therapy for Ethnic Minorities London. Sage publications: 2003.

Systemic approaches

Systemic approaches draw on general systems theory as well as family therapy, to understand communication within families as well as looking at the wider social context. An individual's behaviour is influenced and maintained by how the family members behave towards each other.

Although initially developed for working with families, systemic approaches can also be used with couples.

A genogram or a family tree can provide a useful visual representation of relationships across the generations.

Concepts informing practice

Hypothesizing

This involves using the information available to generate ideas about how a problem is located in the family. It begins with the information contained in the referral, and continues using the behaviour of the family during the session.

Circularity

This is a questioning technique used as part of the interview process, to examine the relationship between people. Family members are asked for their view on how other members relate to each other. This reveals repetitive patterns of behaviour and communication between people. Asking for each person's view helps to engage all the participants.

Neutrality

The concept of neutrality is a pragmatic one that enables the therapist to hear multiple perspectives without taking sides. It is important to prevent any bias, as it is the system, and not any one individual, who is the target of change.

Sessions

Systemic approaches are characterized by team working. Conventionally, this approach uses a one-way screen that separates the therapist and the family from the rest of the team. During a break, the team can feedback their observations and impressions, either to the therapist or directly to the family.

The therapist may give the feedback to the family in the form of 'messages'. These are succinct statements that can be classified as:

- *Supportive* – e.g. commenting positively on communication between the members.
- *Hypothesis-related* – relaying information about members taking up particular roles for the family.
- *Prescriptive* – e.g. giving the family a specific task.

Madeline O'Carroll, City University, London

Further reading

Dallos, R, Draper, R. *An Introduction to Family Therapy*, Open University Press: Buckingham, 2000.

Dialectic Behavioural Therapy (DBT)

DBT was developed following unsuccessful attempts to apply Cognitive Behavioural Therapy (CBT) to a group of young women who all fitted the criteria for diagnosis of borderline personality disorder.

Three sets of strategies and their theories form the three foundations of DBT:

- Validation-acceptance-based strategies help the client see that their thoughts, feelings, and behaviour are 'normal'. This helps them to discover that they have sound judgments and to learn how and when to trust themselves.
- Change-based strategies emphasize to the client that change must occur if they are to build a better life for themselves.
- Dialectic strategies allow the therapist to balance acceptance and change in each session, and enable the sessions to move on with speed, movement and flow. This prevents clients from becoming stuck in rigid thoughts, feelings and behaviours.

Functions and modes

Linehan[1] hypothesized that any successful therapy must have five critical functions:

- Enhance and maintain the client's motivation to change.
- Enhance the client's capabilities.
- Ensure the client's new capabilities are generalized.
- Enhance the therapist's motivation to treat clients, whilst enhancing the therapist's capabilities.
- Structure the environment so the treatment can take place.

The individual therapist maintains the client's motivation for treatment. Clients skills are acquired, developed, strengthened, and generalized through skills training groups, phone coaching, vivo coaching, and homework assignments. Therapists are prevented from burning out by weekly meetings with a consultation team who provide both leadership and support to individual therapists. Therapists and clients meet with families to ensure that adaptive behaviours are being rewarded rather than maladaptive ones reinforced.

Stages and targets

To prevent DBT falling into a treatment that addresses the crisis of the moment week after week, there are targets and stages that are to be followed:

- The first target of the first stage addresses behaviours that could lead to the client's death.
- The second target addresses behaviours that lead to the client stopping treatment.
- The third target is building a better quality of life through the acquisition of new skills.

The second stage is to build on all targets of the first stage. So if the first target was to stop self-harm, the second stage would be to move on

Rosemary Russell, Community Mental Health Team Leader, Perth, West Australia

from quiet desperation to full emotional experiencing. PTSD would be treated in this stage.

The third stage focuses on the problems of living; the goal is that the client has a normal life of happiness and unhappiness.

The fourth stage has to be designed for clients that fail to have a sense of connectedness with a greater whole. The goal is that they develop an ongoing capacity to experience joy and freedom, and that they move away from a sense of incompleteness.

Reference

1 Linehan, M. *Cognitive Behavioural Therapy for Borderline Personality Disorder*. The Guilford Press: New York, 1993.

Further reading

www.behavioraltech.org

Gestalt Therapy

Gestalt therapy is a form of psychotherapy based on the experiential idea of the 'here and now', and on the relationship an individual has with others and their environment. The practice of Gestalt therapy is based on personal experience; an awareness of feelings and behaviour is at its centre. The object is to help the client gain greater independence in their actions and overcome any blockages to their development.

Assumptions

- You cannot work with the mind without taking the body into account – particular emotions are associated with certain postures, for example sad, unhappy, withdrawn are associated with reduced eye contact and barriers such as crossed arms.
- An individual is not aware of the entirety of self – they will only be aware of the role they are in at that point in time e.g. patient, professional, to the exclusion of other roles e.g. mother.
- The mind works on at least two different levels – that which is in the forefront and that which is in the background e.g. pain in the forefront will take priority over all other activities or obligations until resolved.

How the therapist works

- They expose excessive concentration on past events or future plans to focus on what is in the present (actuality).
- They encourage awareness of thoughts, feelings, body posture, breathing rhythm, and physical sensations, thereby enhancing the day-to-day experience (attention).
- They encourage experimentation using dramatization – involving people who are currently significant to the client brought as significant material to the session by the client.
- They replace the concept of blame with the responsibility to create flexibility within relationships.
- They use the five key concepts of awareness:
  - *Contact* – individual interpretation of what is going on as opposed to the perspective of others.
  - *Sensing* – touching feeling, auditory, visual perception (close sensing), thoughts, dreams, body sensations, and emotions (proprioception).
  - *Excitement* – a range of emotional and physiological reactions connecting our senses to what is happening in the immediate environment.
  - *Figure formation* – the way a central focus of interest emerges.
  - *Wholeness* – the holistic approach where the whole is greater than the sum of its parts.

Helen Waldock, Health and Social Care Advisory Service.

Key properties of Gestalt therapy

- *Emergence* – becomes visible or apparent; the 'light bulb' moment.
- *Reification* – treating an abstract concept as if it were real.
- *Multi-stability* – alternating between two or more mutually exclusive states over time e.g. role clarification.
- *Invariance* – developing a quality of being that is resistant to variation, an acceptance of 'you are what you are'.

Further reading

Houston, G. *Brief Gestalt Therapy.* London. Sage Publications: 2003.
Polster, E, Polster, M. *Gestalt Therapy Integrated: contours of theory and practice.* New York. Random House: 1974.

Psychodynamic Therapy

Psychodynamic Therapy is a type of psychoanalytic therapy that aims to help people understand the roots of their emotional distress, often by exploring their unconscious motives, needs, and defences. Simply stated, psychotherapy teaches the client to be honest about their feelings. It is one of several mainstream therapies that focus on aspects of the personality, and it is used to treat a variety of conditions, such as depression and personality disorders. Psychodynamic approaches are centered on the idea of maladapted functions (moods, behaviors, reactions) developed early in life which are at least in part unconscious. Therapy sessions have strict boundaries to preserve the sanctity of the therapeutic hour.

How a psychodynamic therapist works

- The therapist develops a relationship with the client which aims to explore their subconscious mind. In order to do this the therapist must have an in-depth knowledge of themselves as a person to be aware of any counter transference (see below).
- The therapist enables trust and understanding in the therapeutic relationship by first addressing the anxiety associated with the maladaptive function.
- The therapist employs free association and free floating attention involving a great idea of introspection and reflection from the client.
- The therapist reflects how the client is feeling – through words and behaviour – working through resistance and defense mechanisms.
- The therapist uses transference and counter-transference (see below).
- The therapist facilitates insights and understanding through linking the past and the present.
- The therapist interprets the clients' communications as images and descriptions.
- The therapist interprets any transference in terms of past relationships.

There are two key dimensions to psychodynamic therapy:

1. Human development
- Considering the development of individuals from childhood, through adolescence and into adult life, in particular the first 5 to 6 years (formative years).
- Considering past human development in general, and related to the personal history of the client. History taking with the client is an essential initial activity.

2. Personality structure
- Addressing the basic conflicts that can exist between desires and needs.
- Exploring the internalized sense of what is right and what is wrong.
- Acting as a mediator within the demands of the external world e.g. role clarification.
- Challenging the two main defence mechanisms – those which deny reality and those which distort reality.

Helen Waldock, Health and Social Care Advisory Service.

Transference refers to the unconscious tendency of a person to assign to others in the present, those feelings and attitudes originally linked with significant figures in their early life. This might take the form of identifying the therapist with a parent, and may be negative (hostile) or positive (affectionate).

Counter-transference is when the therapist unconsciously begins to transfer their own repressed feelings onto their client.

Further reading

Dryden, W. *Handbook of Individual Therapies.* Sage Publications: London 2002.
Jacobs, M. *Presenting Past: Core of Psychodynamic Counselling and Therapy.* Open University Press: Buckingham, 1998.

Creative Therapies

The creative therapies use artistic interventions and creative processes in therapeutic, rehabilitative, community, and educational settings to promote health, communication, and expression. They aim to foster the integration of physical, emotional, cognitive, and social functioning, to enhance self-awareness, and to facilitate change.

As with all therapies, the relationship between the therapist and the client is of central importance. Creative therapies differ from other psychological therapies because there is a three-way process between the client, the therapist, and the creative process or intervention. These therapies offer an opportunity for expression and communication with people who find it particularly hard to express their thoughts and feelings verbally. All creative therapies should be practiced by trained and qualified therapists.

Creative therapies can be used with individuals, couples, families, and groups.

Art therapy

This involves using art materials for self-expression and reflection in the presence of a trained art therapist. Clients who are referred to an art therapist may not have previous experience or skill in art, as the therapist is not primarily concerned with making an aesthetic assessment of the client's image. The overall aim is to enable the client to change and grow on a personal level, through using affective properties of different art materials in a safe and facilitating environment.

Music therapy

Music therapists use both instrumental and vocal strategies to facilitate changes that are non-musical in their nature. It promotes physical rehabilitation by facilitating movement, increasing motivation to become engaged in treatment, and providing an emotional catharsis and an outlet for expressing feelings. It can also be applied in reminiscence/orientation work with the elderly, through song writing and listening.

Bibliotherapy

Developmental interactive bibliotherapy refers to the use of literature, discussion, and creative writing; it can be used in preventative mental health as well as for assessment, stimulation, and orientation. It promotes understanding, self expression, self-esteem, and interpersonal skills, and can help people find new meaning through new ideas, insights, and information. The use of poetry can be applied to promote self expression, catharsis, and personal growth.

Helen Waldock, Health and Social Care Advisory Service.

Drama therapy

Drama therapy is the systematic and intentional use of processes from drama or theatre, to achieve the therapeutic goals of symptom relief, emotional and physical integration, and personal growth. It is an active approach that allows the client to tell their story, solve a problem, achieve a catharsis, extend the breadth and depth of an inner experience, understand the meaning of images, and strengthen their ability to observe personal roles while increasing flexibility between roles.

Dance therapy

Dance or movement therapy is the use of movement which furthers the emotional, cognitive, and physical integration of an individual. It is based on the assumption that the body and mind are interrelated. It involves direct expression through the body, and is therefore a powerful medium for therapy. This therapy can affect changes in feelings, cognition, physical functioning, and behaviour.

Further reading

Wells, C, Atkinson, K. *Creative Therapies*. Cheltenham. Nelson Thornes: 2000.
Jennings, M. *The Map of Your Mind*. McLelland & Stewart Ltd: Plattsburgh, New York. 2001.

Self-help

Though the term self-help can refer to any case whereby an individual or a group (support group) betters themselves economically, intellectually or emotionally, the connotations of the phrase have come to apply particularly to psychological or psychotherapeutic arenas, often supported through the use of a 'self-help' book, of which there are many.

Rational recovery (RR)

Guidance, and direct instruction on self-recovery from addiction to alcohol and other drugs through planned, permanent abstinence designed as an alternative to Alcoholics Anonymous (AA) 12 step programme (see below). The RR program is based on cognitive behaviour therapy and dissociation from addictive impulses via a website, books, videos, and lectures.

- RR does not regard alcoholism as a disease, but rather a voluntary behaviour.
- RR discourages adoption of the forever 'recovering' drunk persona.
- There are no RR groups.
- Great emphasis is placed on self-efficacy.
- There are no discrete steps and no consideration of religious matters.

The twelve steps

Primary belief of members is that their success is based on giving up on self-reliance and willpower, and instead relying on God, or a 'Higher Power'.

1. Admit we were powerless over alcohol; that our lives have become unmanageable.
2. Come to believe that a power greater than ourselves could restore sanity.
3. Make a decision to turn our will and our lives over to the care of God as we understand Him.
4. Make a searching and fearless moral inventory of ourselves.
5. Admit to God, to ourselves, and to another human being the exact nature of our wrongs.
6. Be entirely ready to have God remove all our defects of character.
7. Humbly ask God to remove our shortcomings.
8. Make a list of all persons we have harmed, and be willing to make amends to them.
9. Make direct amends to such people wherever possible, except when to do so would injure them or others.
10. Continue to take personal inventory and when we are wrong promptly admit it.
11. Seek through prayer and meditation to improve our conscious contact with God, as we understand Him.
12. Having had a spiritual awakening this message is carried to alcoholics and the principles practised these in all their affairs.

(Source: Alcoholics Anonymous)

Professor Dave Richards, University of York.

Critics of these programmes, however, often hold that this reliance is ineffective, and offensive or inapplicable to atheists and others who do not believe in a God.

Supporting self-help

Supporting people in using self-help is critical to its effectiveness. Self-help materials may have less benefit without some form of support and guidance, although some computerized self-help programmes mimic a therapist's behaviour and are effective with minimal-guidance.

In guided self-help (GSH), nurses should be extremely familiar with the materials they are supporting. Therapeutic contacts will be brief, and sometimes on the telephone, so nurses should be highly skilled in developing a rapid therapeutic alliance, initially engaging people and then developing and maintaining that alliance, despite the brevity of contact. It is more effective to have short but frequent contacts than to have a few long contacts.

Self-help should be situated within a 'stepped care' system Although it may be useful for some people, others who are not improving will need 'stepping up' to traditional psychological therapy or psychiatric care. Decisions about stepping up should be the result of a scheduled review, supported by standardized outcome measures, where the nurse and client can discuss the next stage of a shared plan.

Further reading

Lovell, K, Richards, DA, Bower, P. Improving access to primary care mental health: uncontrolled evaluation of a pilot self-help clinic. British *Journal of General Practice* **53**: 133–5, 2003.

National Institute for Health and Clinical Excellence. Depression: management of depression in primary and secondary care, Clinical Guideline 23. NIHCE: London, 2004.

Complementary therapies

These are therapies that are not part of orthodox medical treatment; they are not usually administered by a medically trained practitioner and are not normally available in a traditional hospital setting (*but some, like acupuncture, are available in NHS hospitals by qualified practitioners who may or may not be medically trained*). Complementary therapies can be used alongside or instead of traditional medicine. However, some of these treatments can interact with traditional medicine; this can sometimes cause complications. Complementary therapies should only be administered by a practitioner who is fully trained in that particular therapy, following a comprehensive health assessment.

Complementary therapies have been used for many centuries, and some of these treatments are the foundations of the traditional medicines we use today.

Herbalism

Herbs have been used since the dawn of time as medicines and many common drugs are made from herbal extracts. The natural chemical properties of certain herbs have been shown to contain medicinal value. However, unlike conventional medicine, herbalists use the 'whole' herb or plant rather than isolating and breaking down chemical compounds and then synthesising them into compounds. This is because the plant, being a part of nature, is said to represent perfect balance; healing requires the natural combination of elements in the plant or herb, not just a single chemical within it.

Homeopathy

Homeopathy was developed in 18th century by Samuel Hahemann (1753–1843). It is based on the belief that 'like cures like'. Remedies are derived from plants, animals and minerals. These are diluted and given in minute doses. The idea is that the same substance that that causes symptoms if given to a healthy person can be used in much smaller doses to cure the unwell. For example, caffeine given to healthy person causes central nervous system stimulation and increased urine output. Caffeine given in much smaller doses could be used in homeopathy for someone complaining of excess urine, sleeplessness, and unusual mental activity.

Homeopathy strives to treat the cause of the illness not the symptoms thus preventing a reoccurrence of illness.

Reiki

Reiki was developed in Japan by Dr Usui and brought to the west in 1930s. It is a gentle non-invasive technique, based on channelling energy through seven major chakras or energy centers in the body to treat physical and emotional ailments. The practitioner does not touch their client, but moves their hands a few centimetres above the body, slowly moving over the entire body. They detect the areas of heat which are the areas needing treatment. Opening up the chakras allows the energy meridians to flow and balances the body's energy, restoring a healthy aura, and thus a healthy body.

Rosemary Russell, Community Mental Health Team Leader, Perth, West Australia.

Reflexology

This is the technique of applying gentle pressure to reflexes in both hands and feet. These reflexes correspond to particular parts of the body. When stimulated, these parts of the nervous system invoke responses in the relevant parts of the body to promote a feeling of deep relaxation; the subsequent restoration of balance in the body brings healing. Balance can be lost through prolonged stress and illness.

Acupuncture

Acupuncture is based on a belief in Chinese and Eastern medicine of a motivating energy source called 'Qi'. This energy source needs to be able to move through the body in a balanced, smooth way through a series of meridians or chakras under the skin. When the flow of energy is unbalanced, illness ensues. By inserting fine needles into the channels of energy, the acupuncturist can stimulate the body's own healing process. This achieves physical, emotional, and spiritual balance in the individual.

Shiatsu

This is a Japanese technique of massage, based on similar principles of using the energy flow or meridians in the body. The Shiatsu practitioner uses a series of gentle holding, pressing with palms, thumbs, elbows, knees, and feet on the meridians. When appropriate more dynamic rotations and stretches are used. Once energy flow is restored, good health follows.

Further reading

Nurses Handbook of Alternative and Complementary Therapies. Springhouse Lippincott Williams & Wilkins: 2002.

Psychosocial interventions for psychoses

Psychosocial interventions for psychoses, including those psychoses in schizophrenia, involves a combination of drug treatment, other therapies and treatments, plus ongoing support and rehabilitation strategies. These include case management, family intervention for carers, cognitive behavioural therapy, social skills training, and psycho-education.

History of psychosocial interventions

The introduction of antipsychotic medication for schizophrenia in the 1950s led to a belief that the symptoms of the illness could be eliminated by the use of these drugs.

Alongside this, changes in the understanding of mental illness led to changes in mental health policy in the United States and in the United Kingdom. The result was the large-scale closure of psychiatric beds and the loss of 'asylum' (place of refuge or sanctuary for the mentally ill). Responsibility and care for the mentally ill was placed firmly with the family and community.

Unfortunately drug treatment was wholly effective for only 30% of patients. Many patients who did not significantly recover with medication continued to experience residual psychotic symptoms, and were at risk of a relapse of the illness.

Schizophrenia can be a chronic lifetime illness for up to 60% of patients. Since the early 1970s, researchers have investigated the impact of psychosocial factors and effective interventions on the course of the illness.

Relapse is a common feature of schizophrenia and is characterized by a resurgence of symptoms, consequent distress, loss of hope, and a further reduction of social function and role. A person's vulnerability to relapse can be both in-born (genetic) and acquired (as a result of life events). Relapse is most likely to occur when street drugs are used, when drug treatment is inadequate or stopped spontaneously, stressful family situations, stigma, social isolation, or as a consequence of chaotic admissions to hospital. Psychosocial interventions aim to reduce the distress caused by active symptoms, reduce the frequency and impact of relapse, improve social function and improve quality of life.

Types of psychosocial interventions

Case management

Case management ensures that mental health professionals work collaboratively with service users to deliver areas of care and rehabilitation. This model underpins current assertive outreach interventions, by enabling the service user to remain in control of their treatment via the Care Programme Approach.

Jan Murray, East London and the City Mental Health NHS Trust.

Family work

Patients returning to environments of high expressed emotion (where carers use criticism of the patient, are emotionally over-involved and have unrealistic expectations of the patient, their treatment, and prognosis and rehabilitation goals) were twice as likely to relapse within the first nine months following discharge. Family work developed from these studies; it aims to provide assessment, information giving, problem solving techniques and interventions to reduce stress for carers.

Cognitive behavioural therapy (CBT)

Despite psychotropic medication, 30–40% of patients will relapse while on medication, and a significant number will continue to experience positive symptoms. The aim of cognitive behavioural therapy is to reduce the impact of these symptoms, by reducing distress, dysfunctional beliefs, feelings and behaviours. A range of techniques are used including: coping strategy enhancement, psycho-education, interventions to reduce associated anxiety and mood problems, and goal setting.

📖 Cognitive Behavioural Therapy

Further reading

Berke, JH. Beyond Madness: Psychosocial Interventions in Psychosis. London. Jessica Kingsley Publishing: 2001.

Harris, N. Psychosocial interventions for People with Schizophrenia: a practice guide for mental health workers. London. Palgrave Macmillan: 2002.

Behavioural activation

Behavioural activation (BA) is a structured psychological treatment for depression. Its theoretical basis is that depression is best understood as a functional problem, and that altering the external context rather than internal factors (such as a person's thoughts) is likely to lead to improvement.

Behavioural theory considers that the behaviours associated with depression lead to a reduction in opportunities for people to experience pleasure (positive reinforcement), whilst rewarding avoidance (negative reinforcement). When depression strikes, people withdraw from situations and activities that give them negative feelings, and they find it increasingly harder to return to these activities. This reduces the possibility that they will have pleasant experiences. Depressive behaviours make depression worse.

Treatment

Although behavioural activation is often used in cognitive behavioural therapy (CBT) as the first stage of treatment, research trials have shown that when BA is used as a stand-alone treatment, it is just as effective as CBT, cognitive therapy or antidepressants. BA is also the essential component of problem solving treatment for depression, and has been used successfully in many collaborative care and self-help trials.

Essentially, BA targets avoidance behaviour. It identifies activities which a depressed person has reduced in their lives. These can be categorized into routine, pleasurable, and necessary activities. Routine activities are those things we do, often mundane, which 'anchor' our lives – activities such as shopping, cleaning, cooking, and getting up at the same time every day. Pleasurable activities include private leisure (e.g. reading the newspaper) and social pursuits (e.g. talking to friends). Necessary activities are often aversive, for example, dealing with a conflict at work, paying bills, filling in forms.

People start behavioural activation by coming up with three separate lists of routine, pleasurable, and necessary activities. They then make a hierarchal list of a mixture of all three types of activities from easiest to hardest. Finally, activities are selected from low down the list and weekly plans developed to reactivate them. Each week, the diaries are reviewed and new activities scheduled.

Supporting behavioural activation

Nurses and other mental health professionals can support patients using behavioural activation. It is easy to teach, and highly acceptable to patients and workers. Telephone support can often be effective, provided some face-to-face education sessions and good quality information manuals have been provided previously.

Professor Dave Richards, University of York.

Further reading

Hopko, DR, Lejuez, CW, Ruggiero, KJ, et al. Contemporary behavioral activation treatments for depression: Procedures, principles, and progress. *Clinical Psychology Review* **23**: 699–717, 2003.
Jacobson, NS, Martell, CR, Dimidjian, S. Behavioral activation therapy for depression: returning to contextual roots. *Clinical Psychology: Science and Practice* **8**(3): 255–70, 2001.

Relapse prevention

Relapse prevention in mental health falls into three areas: pharmacological, psychological, and combination approaches. Combination approaches are the preferred option.

Pharmacological relapse prevention

At least 45% of people diagnosed with schizophrenia and bipolar affective disorder do not take their medication as prescribed. This problem is not unique to individuals suffering from mental health problems; non-compliance with medication is found at similar levels in the treatment of tuberculosis, diabetes, and leprosy.

Non-compliance with medication is thought to increase the possibility of relapse in schizophrenia by at least a factor of 4. In bipolar affective disorder, non-compliance with medication is the most robust predictor of subsequent hospital admission, considerably above all other causative factors.

Pharmacological relapse prevention shares many of the fundamental precepts of medication management (see topic medicines management). Any medication prescription regime that aims to prevent relapse through medication non-compliance should be a result of a decision made between the prescriber, the service user and any mental health practitioner who is in close regular contact with the service user. This will reduce the non-compliance that results from matters such as side-effects of medication, health beliefs, and cultural preferences.

Factors relevant to pharmacological relapse prevention include:
• The joint planning of a medication regime.
• Suitability of the prescribed medication profile.
• Analysis of barriers to adherence and problem solving.
• Motivational interviewing to eradicate or reduce these barriers.

Psychological relapse prevention

Research consistently shows that even when service users are fully compliant with medication, breakthrough episodes of illness are the norm. Medication alone is thought to prevent relapse in only 30–50% of individuals with a psychotic disorder, and the figures are similar in mood disorders.

It is clear that relapse prevention based solely on promoting adherence to medication is insufficient for at least half of all service users: psychological strategies aimed at minimizing relapse are equally important.

There are a number of models of psychological relapse prevention, and central to each is the concept of prodrome management. The word prodrome is derived from the Greek word 'prodromos' which means the forerunner of an event.

Paul Hammersly, University of Manchester

Prodrome management or early warning signs management

Service users are encouraged to identify individual early signs that an illness episode may be imminent. These signs may be physical (sleeplessness), behavioural (a change in behavioural routine), affective (emergence of mood associated with illness episode), or cognitive (alteration in cognitive mechanisms such as appraisal of danger). Prodromes vary between individuals but tend to be consistent for each individual.

Prodrome recognition therapy

Service users are asked to identify their own early warning signs, often from a list or card sort.[2] This list is then refined, often with the help of family, friends or mental health workers. Early signs are then ranked, according to at which point in an episode they occur – at the start, middle or end. Once the prodrome list has been established, an action plan is devised detailing what action should be taken when a prodrome is identified, to prevent the onset of a full episode of illness.

Each action plan is individual to the needs of the service user, and may include factors such as behavioural change, change to medication or the promotion of awareness of cognitive biases or misinterpretations. The promotion of assistance-seeking on identification of a prodrome is particularly important.

Combined approaches

Combined approaches are simply the combination of pharmacological and psychological relapse prevention plans, and are in most cases the preferred option.

Reference

2 Perry, A; Tarrier, N, Morriss, R, McCarthy, E. and Limb, K. Randomized controlled trial of the efficacy of teaching patients with bipolar disorder to identify early symptoms of relapse and obtain treatment. *British Medical Journal* **318**: 139–53, 1999.

Further reading

McPhillips, M, Sensky, T. Coercion, adherence or collaboration? Influences on compliance with medication. In: T Wykes et al. (eds.) *Outcome and Innovation in the psychological treatment of schizophrenia*. Wiley: London 1998.

Assertive outreach teams

Client group

Assertive outreach teams (AOT) aim to meet the needs of people with high levels of disability associated with severe and persistent mental health problems such as schizophrenia. Typically, users of assertive outreach services have a history of frequent inpatient use and complex multiple needs; including the risk of self-harm, persistent offending, substance use or insecure accommodation. Most assertive outreach service users have a history of difficulties in maintaining lasting and consenting contact with services.

Team purpose

These teams initially focus on engagement, by providing ongoing support to the client, their carer, or their family. As therapeutic alliances develop, they aim to reduce hospital admissions, lengths of stay, and symptom severity and to improve social functioning.

Assertive outreach is not an intervention in itself, but it is a platform from which interventions are delivered. A future challenge for AO teams is the integration of vocational, employment and other socially rehabilitative interventions into existing service provision.

'Assertive' implies a tenacious and persistent approach rather than an aggressive one, emphasizing the need for creative interventions that foster engagement.

Team characteristics and principles

Assertive outreach teams differ in terms of size, staff composition and the service sector in which they are based. They originate from within mainstream psychiatry, but an increasing number now operate from the voluntary sector. Differences between statutory and voluntary sector services are often unclear. Voluntary sector services tend not to hold formal clinical responsibility, they are smaller, contain fewer staff disciplines, and have no control over inpatient bed usage.

Recommended principles of assertive outreach care include:
- A self-contained service responsible for a wide range of interventions.
- A single responsible medical officer as an active team member.
- A long-term treatment emphasizing continuity of care.
- Most services delivered in community settings.
- Ongoing contact and relationship-building with service users.
- Overall care coordination responsibility.
- Small caseloads of no more than 12 clients per worker.

Iain Ryrie, Assistant Director of Research, Mental Health Foundation

Outcomes

Assertive outreach teams have been remarkably successful in engaging users, many of whom report satisfaction with services. Beneficial health outcomes have also been reported, although the teams have yet to make significant and long lasting contributions to individuals' social functioning.

Further reading

Burns, T, Firn, M. *Assertive Outreach in Mental Health: A Manual for Practitioners.* Oxford University Press: Oxford, 2002.
Department of Health. The Mental Health Policy Implementation Guide. DoH: London, 2001.

Early intervention in psychosis

An early recognition of psychosis allows early intervention and the initiation of appropriate treatment and management strategies. Delays can have serious consequences for patients and families.

Benefits of early intervention

Studies of early intervention demonstrate that it reduces the risk of people developing a florid psychosis. In addition, with early intervention they may experience:

- More rapid recovery.
- Better prognosis.
- Preservation of psychosocial skills.
- Preservation of family and social supports.
- Maintenance of social and educational status.
- Decreased need for hospitalization.
- More effective treatment within the 'critical period' (see 'Risks' opposite).
- Reduced duration of untreated illness.

Epidemiology of psychosis

The risk factors for psychotic illness include old age, adolescence and young adulthood. They also include existing traits or vulnerabilities such as:

- Family history of mental illness.
- Vulnerable personality (e.g. schizoid personality type).
- Delayed milestones (walking, talking).
- Low intelligence.
- History of obstetric or perinatal complications.
- Winter birth.
- Stress factors including: life events, perceived psychosocial stress, substance misuse, subjective or functional changes.

History of early intervention in psychosis

Delays in treatment result in significant distress for patients, as well as incomplete recovery, poorer prognosis, higher suicide risk, substance misuse, and enduring levels of social disability. Delays in receiving treatment are independently associated with a greatly increased risk of relapse.

'Prodrome' has been identified as a period of non-psychotic disturbance that occurs just before the emergence of a psychotic episode. If the patient is left undiagnosed and untreated they will go on to develop a psychotic illness. If prodrome can be recognized, and treatment offered, it may be possible to divert the progression to a psychotic illness. Delays in treatment of up to a year have been reported. These delays are often characterized by unavailable care pathways and signs going unrecognized.

Jan Murray, East London and the City Mental Health NHS Trust

Clinical features of prodrome or a pre-psychotic state

Adolescents and young adults are in a highly transitory life stage. However, the persistent presence of the following signs over a two week period should arouse a suspicion that the patient may be in an 'at risk' mental state:

- Suspiciousness
- Depression
- Anxiety and tension
- Irritability
- Anger
- Mood swings
- Sleep disturbances
- Appetite changes
- Loss of energy or motivation
- Perception that things around them have altered
- Belief that things have sped up or slowed down
- Deterioration in work or study
- Lack of interest in socializing
- Emergence of unusual beliefs e.g. magical thinking.

These signs may be present in stress and other disorders. An unexplained loss of social function or a sustained lack of contact with peers should further arouse suspicion.

Principles of early intervention

These include:

- Treatment of psychotic symptoms with low dose atypical anti-psychotic medication.
- Treatment of accompanying anxiety or depression.
- Gaining the patient's trust, promote compliance with antipsychotic treatment (psycho-education).
- Making an effort to minimize distress associated with hospitalization and treatment.
- Involving family and friends in recovery plan. Being mindful of the phasic nature of the illness, and using a staged approach.

Risks

One in five young men with adolescent onset schizophrenia commits suicide. 70% of young suicides involve substance misuse. The critical period from the onset of psychoses to schizophrenia is between 2–5 years. An inadequate and untimely treatment period increases the duration of untreated psychoses. This leads to increased risk of relapse, residual symptoms, social disability, and reduced quality of life.

Further reading

Edwards, J, McGorry, P. *Implementing Early Intervention in Psychosis*. Martia Dunitz 2002.

Group Therapy

Group therapy is an intervention in which between 8 and 10 people meet together to discuss issues that cause them concern.

The aims of group therapy

Group therapy gives members an opportunity to:
- Try out new ways of behaving.
- Learn more about the way they interact with others.
- Share their feelings and thoughts in an open and honest manner.
- Develop trust in working with others.
- Learn how to work with others.
- Receive feedback from others on how they relate to others.
- Interact freely with others.
- Resolve the issues that led them to seeking help.
- Provide support to, and receive support from, others.
- Help themselves and others find healthy alternatives to troubling issues.
- Develop new skills in relating to people.

Indications for group therapy

Group therapy is indicated for people who:
- Wish to explore issues in a context that is closer to real life.
- Welcome the opportunity to reflect on their own and others' interpersonal skills.
- Will benefit from active participation with others.
- Want feedback from others on issues that are troubling them.
- Have deficits in their interpersonal and social skills.
- Have problems developing trust in working with others.
- Want to learn more about how they interact with others.
- Want to learn more about how they relate to others.

Patrick Callaghan, Professor of Mental Health Nursing, University of Nottingham & Nottinghamshire Healthcare NHS Trust

The effectiveness of group therapy

There is evidence from well-designed studies that group therapy leads to successful outcomes for people living with mental health problems including depression, anorexia nervosa, schizophrenia, alcohol dependency, and suicidal adolescents.

Further reading

Roth, A, Fonagy, P. *What Works for Whom? A critical review of psychotherapy research*, 2nd edn. The Guilford Pres: New York, 2004.

Rutgers College Counselling Centre. Group Therapy Virtual Brochure. Available at: www.rci.rutgers.edu

Joint crisis plans for people with psychosis

Joint Crisis Plans (JCPs) are a collaborative means of working that are developed between mental health teams and service users. The aim is for the service user and the clinical team to reach agreement, through negotiation and consensus building.

Each completed crisis card or plan has information, an assessment of past crises, as well as an advance plan for care in a crisis. JCPs have psychological value for the carrier/holder and they are a potential advocacy tool for use during a crisis.

A joint crisis plan agreement is achieved prior to any episode of illness, and at a time when the service user is well enough to develop a crisis plan. JCPs (carried by the service user) are thought to be especially useful during a crisis, when individuals may be too unwell to articulate any treatment preferences.

This approach has been likened to the advance directives and living wills referred to within the literature on physical illness.[3]

There is a high rate of relapse among people suffering from psychosis. This may result in numerous admissions to inpatient psychiatric units, and it is distressing for the individuals concerned. JCPs aim to mitigate some of the negative consequences of relapse including admission to hospital, the use of coercion in the form of the application of the Mental Health Act, and the costs associated with these consequences.

Henderson et al. showed that JCPs were able to significantly reduce compulsory in-patient treatment, compared with treatment as usual.[4] JCP users experienced fewer admissions and a significantly reduced use of the Mental Health Act. 13% experienced compulsory admission or treatment, compared with 27% of the control group.

Advance directives in the form of the JCP approach have the potential to impact positively by reducing containment and costs. There is a strong case for selecting the JCP approach as an intervention and for their inclusion in policy making.

Included in a JCP are examples of the paperwork used to elicit user preferences as well as an example of a completed crisis plan.

📖 Relapse prevention

Chris Flood, City University, London

References

3 Stewart, K, Bowker L. Advance directives and living wills. *Postgrad Med J* **74** (869):151–6, 1998.
4 Henderson, C, Flood C, Leese, M, et al. Effect of joint crisis plans on use of compulsory treatment in psychiatry: single blind randomized controlled trial. *British Medical Journal* **317**: 1195–2000, 2004.

Six category intervention analysis

Six category intervention analysis is a communication/counselling framework developed by John Heron. It is a tool for nurses to select, monitor, and reflect on their communication skills and interactions with their clients. It provides a way of classifying a huge range of skills under six types of interventions which include six kinds of purpose or intention. These intentions underlie the ultimate choice of intervention and can be applied equally to one-to-one and group communications.

Interventions

Six categories and their designations are either Authoritative or Facilitative.

Authoritative interventions are so called because in each case the practitioner is taking a more overtly dominant or assertive role. The emphasis is more on what the practitioner is doing and includes:

1. Prescriptive: aims to direct the behaviour of the client. For example, to give advice – *'I think you will feel better if you talk about why you are anxious.'*

2. Informative: aims to impart new knowledge and information to the client. For example to give information – *'These tablets can cause you to feel drowsy'*.

3. Confronting: aims to directly challenge the restrictive attitude/belief/behaviour of the client. For example to challenge or give direct feedback –*'Are you aware that when you shout you frighten your family?'*

Facilitative interventions are less obtrusive and more discreet while the emphasis is on the effect of the intervention on the client.

4. Cathartic: aims to enable the client to abreact painful emotion. For example to help release tensions or encourage laughter/crying – *'From what you have experienced – I can imagine how angry you may feel'*.

5.. Catalytic: aims to enable the client to learn and develop by self-direction and self discovery within the context of practitioner-client situation, but also beyond it. For example encourage self-directed problem solving – *'How do you think you could improve your situation?'*

6. Supportive: aims to affirm the worth and value of the client. For example – be approving/validating – *'You really tried to control your anger.'*

Each of the six categories is value neutral with no one category being more or less important than the other when used in an appropriate context. However, they are only of real value if rooted in care and concern for the client's sake.

Jean Morrissey, Trinity College, Dublin

Applying six category intervention analysis

In practice, the skill of the nurse is to be:
- Equally proficient in each of the six categories.
- Aware of which category s/he is using and why at any given time.
- Able to move skillfully from one type of intervention to any other as the developing situation and purpose of the interaction requires.

Further reading

Ashmore, R, Banks, D. Student Nurses' use of their interpersonal skills with clinical role plays. *Nurse Education Today* **24**(10): 20–9, 2003.

Heron, J. Helping the Client – *A Creative Practical Guide*, 5th edn. Sage Publications: London, 2001.

Sloan, G, Watson, H. John Heron Six Category Intervention Analysis: Towards Understanding interpersonal relations and progressing the delivery of clinical supervision for mental health nursing in the United Kingdom. *Journal of Advanced Nursing* **36**(2): 206–14, 2001.

An intervention to reduce absconding from acute psychiatric wards

Patients who abscond from acute psychiatric wards evoke anxiety in staff, relatives, and carers. Returning the patient to hospital takes up valuable staff and police time. Those close to the patient may lose faith in psychiatric services, and importantly, the patient may deteriorate through loss of contact with psychiatric services.

An intervention package

Research on absconding by Bowers et al. in 1999 provided a basis for the formulation of an intervention package that staff could use to reduce absconding by patients from their wards.[1]

The intervention was tested in a 'before and after' trial in five acute psychiatric wards in 2003. Absconding rates fell by 25% overall during the intervention period. The researchers trained the ward staff in the intervention, which is outlined as follows:

Elements of the intervention
- The use of a signing in and out book so that staff know the location of users.
- Identification of users at high risk of absconding.
- Purposeful nursing time with the identified high-risk group.
- Breaking bad news carefully to these patients.
- Debriefing following ward incidents.
- A multidisciplinary review following two absconds.

Prior to the commencement of the project, the previous research findings and the intervention was explained to staff by the researchers. The benefits of participation for them, as well as for their patients was explained. This dialogue enabled joint working to identify ways in which the intervention could be implemented. The staff also agreed to collect outcome data.

Outcome data
- Data on the frequency of door locking was collected.
- Data on ward incidents was collected with the aid of the Staff Observation Aggression Scale[2].
- Data on the time of absconds was collected.

The intervention commenced on two wards. The staff required considerable support and encouragement, both in data collection and in implementing the package. After a cooling off period the other three wards were supported in implementing the package. At the end of the research, staff were invited to discuss their experiences during participation in focus groups.

Dr Jane Alexander, City University, London

Three wards implemented the intervention successfully, and absconding fell in two of them. For various reasons associated with ward stability, the other two wards did not implement the intervention consistently. Staff on all wards became much more aware of the antecedents to absconding events. Anecdotally, several staff perceived that the ward nursing regimes had become less custodial and more therapeutic as a result of the intervention.

References

1 Bowers, L, Jarrett, M, Clark, N, et al. Absconding: why patients leave. *Journal of Psychiatric and Mental Health Nursing* **6**: 199–205, 1999.
2 Nijman, H, Muris, H, Merckelbach, L, *et al.* The staff observation Scale revised (SOAS-R). *Aggressive Behaviour* **25**(3): 197–203, 1999.

Further reading

Bowers, L, Alexander, J, Gaskell, K. A trial of an anti-absconding intervention in acute psychiatric wards. *Journal of Psychiatric and Mental Health Nursing* **10**: 410–16, 2003.

Violence

Recognizing violence

Violence risk assessment has two main timescales:
- **Short-term** prediction of the likelihood of imminent violence (i.e. hours or minutes).
- **Long-term** prediction (i.e. days, months, or years).

Types of aggression

A useful distinction is between reactive ('hot', emotional) and proactive ('cold', instrumental) aggression; although there is much overlap.

Reactive aggression is a response to an identifiable, proximal trigger or provocation. It has the primary aim of harming the person or the object associated with the trigger; it is largely unplanned and is accompanied by signs of high autonomic system arousal and loss of control.

Proactive aggression is a more planned response in the absence of immediate provocation or high arousal. It has the primary aim of achieving a specific goal (e.g. escape or power) other than direct harm to the targeted person.

Assessment of potential violence

This assessment relies both on close monitoring of the person's behaviour, and on engaging with them from admission onwards. It should take place in the context of understanding the person's background and personal triggers, and within a therapeutic relationship. The most useful predictor is the person's history of previous violence, and the triggers associated with such violence.

Much aggression in mental health services is reactive, occurring in response to perceived provocations. Indicators of angry arousal and potential loss of control in humans include:
- Shouting
- Glaring
- Swearing
- Verbal abuse
- Verbal threats
- Unclear or confused thinking
- Intimidation
- Use of the body (including intrusive gestures)
- Restlessness.

Certain additional predictors are specifically linked to mental disorder, especially evidence of delusions or hallucinations with a violent content. Presence of these behaviours indicates an elevated risk of imminent violence.

People have individual patterns of behaviour; these signals do not indicate that violence is inevitable, nor does the absence of them automatically indicate a low risk of imminent violence. Some acts of aggression occur following a period of withdrawal and silence. The key observation

Dr Richard Whittington, University of Liverpool

to make is to notice any rapid change in behaviour from the person's norm, and to be aware of current stressors or provocations.

Instruments for assessing violence risk
Brøset Violence Checklist (BVC)
Violence Risk Appraisal Guide (VRAG)

Almvik, R, Woods, P. Short-term risk prediction: the Brøset Violence Checklist. *Journal of Psychiatric and Mental Health Nursing* **10**: 231–8, 2003.
Harris, G, Rice, M, Camillen, J. Applying a forensic actuarial assessment (the Violence Risk Appraisal Guide) to non-forensic patients. *Journal of Interpersonal Violence* **19**(9): 1063–74, 2004.

Preventing violence

Once the potential risk has been established, there is much that can be done to reduce the likelihood of violence occurring.

Organizationally

At the organizational level, the physical and the human environment can be improved (for example, ward sightlines, the skill mix of staff, the staff-patient ratio). Training for staff and individualized risk assessment and activity programmes for patients can also be developed. A culture of service user collaboration and involvement should be fostered.

Individually

At the individual level, as soon as possible after admission, the service user should be involved with the staff in identifying their own personal anger triggers and their preferred staff responses. This may be done using an advance directive. (📖 Joint Crisis Plans for People with Psychosis).

Preventative intervention

The interactional level becomes important once violence is judged to be imminent. Three main types of preventative intervention are available: enhanced observation and engagement; de-escalation; and preventative pharmacotherapy.

Enhanced observation and engagement

General observation of inpatients can be enhanced to intermittent (15 minute) checks, observation, and beyond that, to 'within eyesight' and 'within arms length' levels, as the risk escalates. Observation should involve active engagement of the observing staff with the service user at all times.

De-escalation

De-escalation is a set of verbal and non-verbal skills used by staff to reduce the service user's level of angry arousal.

De-escalation skills include:
- Establishing rapport through demonstration of attentiveness, concern, and empathy.
- Reflection and active listening.
- Using open questions.
- Negotiation and encouraging a sense of cooperation.
- Modelling calmness.

Dr Richard Whittington, University of Liverpool

It may include therapeutic limit-setting and instructing, especially for proactive aggression, although this is likely to increase anger in the short term.

De-escalation techniques include:
- Identifying the source of the person's anger.
- Explaining the reasons for perceived provocations.
- Suggesting alternatives.
- Reminders of time, place, and persons involved in the interaction.
- Non-verbal indicators of interest, concern (e.g. head nodding), and personal calmness (e.g. relaxed posture).

Unnecessary proximity, touching, and a hectoring tone of voice should not be used.

Preventative pharmacotherapy
This involves persuading (not coercing, although the line is hard to draw) the service user to accept low levels of tranquillizing medication orally. Medications include haloperidol, lorazepam, olanzapine, and risperidone.

Further reading

Cowin, L, Davies, R, Estall, G, et al. De-escalating Aggression and Violence in the Mental Health Setting. International Journal of Mental Health Nursing 12(1): 64–73, 2003.

National Institute for Clinical Excellence. Violence: The Short-Term Management of Disturbed/violent Behaviour in In-patient Psychiatric Settings and Emergency Department, Clinical Guideline 25. NICE: London, 2005.

Therapeutic management of violence

Effective prediction and prevention will avoid most, but not all, incidents developing into overt violence. If prevention is judged to be failing, and the only alternative available is to manage the threat, therapeutic management may be used. This is likely to include some element of coercion.

Principles

The level of coercion used must be proportionate to the threat presented by the person, and any coercion should be ended as soon as possible, without compromising safety. Potential non-coercive alternatives should be considered at all times.

Explicit policies guiding the use of coercive interventions and recording mechanisms must be in place. Positive engagement and the de-escalation activities (🕮 Preventing violence) must continue alongside coercive interventions, but the potential for negotiation is much reduced at this stage.

There are three main techniques for the therapeutic management of violence: restraint, seclusion, and rapid tranquillization.

Physical (manual) restraint

Physical restraint is used for the immediate emergency management of violence. It involves holding the person and preventing movement. A standing position should be maintained if at all possible, as restraint on the floor can be highly dangerous, and direct pressure on certain parts of the body (e.g. the thorax) can be fatal. A team member should be responsible for supporting the head and neck, ensuring that the person's airway and breathing are not compromised, and monitoring vital signs.

Seclusion

Seclusion involves the enforced segregation of a person in a bare room or an area separate from the ward community. The exit from this room is either locked or blocked by allocated staff. Observation and engagement should be maintained throughout the seclusion period.

Many authorities view seclusion as the most anti-therapeutic of the coercive interventions, and active steps to police it and to reduce its use are being taken worldwide. Some argue for mechanical restraint as an acceptable alternative.

Dr Richard Whittington, University of Liverpool

Rapid tranquillization

This involves the administration of tranquillizing medication. This may have to be done intramuscularly or intravenously while the person is held in restraint. Negotiated acceptance of oral medication may be possible as an alternative, and should be considered on the 'least coercion' principle. Medications given include haloperidol and lorazepam. Observation, and where possible engagement, should be maintained throughout the sedation period.

Throughout this process *of managing violence* the needs of other service users should be considered by allocating at least one staff member to support them if necessary.

Further reading

National Institute for Clinical Excellence. Violence: The Short-Term Management of Disturbed/ violent Behaviour in In-patient Psychiatric Settings and Emergency Department, Clinical Guideline 25. NICE: London, 2005.

Sailas, E, Wahlbeck, K. Restraint and seclusion in psychiatric inpatient wards. *Current Opinion in Psychiatry* **18**(5): 555–9, 2005.

Post-violence incident analysis and management

Once the immediate crisis is resolved, and a safe environment has been restored, the aftermath of a violent incident must be managed, including efforts to learn from the experience. All service users and staff who were directly involved in or witnessed the incident should be considered.

The first priority is to assess and manage any physical injury sustained by any person as a result of the incident. Physical injury may be treated locally or may require referral to an emergency department.

The second priority is to assess and minimize the psychological distress of those staff and service users directly and indirectly involved in the incident. Immediate reassurance and explanations should be provided as appropriate.

Report or post-incident review

A report

A brief, structured report on all violent incidents should be made by the lead person involved, as soon as possible afterwards. This report should follow a template used throughout the organization, and could be based on widely used forms e.g. the Staff Observation of Aggression Scale (SOAS-R).[1] Electronic reporting will expedite communication and review.

Post-incident review

This is more formal than a report. It involves staff, service users and others as appropriate, and should be conducted within 72 hours of the incident. It aims to identify individual support needs and to inform future practice.

Those identified as having significant distress as a result of the incident may require sickness absence, and a phased, supported return to work with service users, over one to two weeks or longer.

Lessons for improved practice are gained through incident analysis. This involves discussion of the relevant warning signs and triggers preceding the incident, and the effectiveness of any physical and psychological techniques used to manage the violence. The role of the environment in the incident should also be considered. The tone of this review should be neutral and non-blaming and, where possible, it should be conducted by somebody not directly involved.

Dr Richard Whittington, University of Liverpool

A collaborative review with the relevant service user is also recommended, to minimize damage to the therapeutic relationship. Action points identified from the review should be incorporated into individual care plans and unit policies. If incidents occur regularly, teams should consider a weekly or monthly review to identify any regular patterns, and should act to incorporate these into care plans and risk assessments for individual service users.

Institutional post-incident reviews by senior staff should also be conducted regularly – these are based on the incident reports, and aim to identify patterns across units and to develop an action plan.

Reference

1 Nijman, HLI, Palmstierna, T, Almvik, R, et al. Fifteen years of research with the Staff Observation Aggression Scale: a review. *Acta Psychiatrica Scandinavica* **111**(1): 12–21, 2005.

Further reading

Flannery, RB Jr. The Assaulted Staff Action Program (ASAP): Ten year empirical support for Critical Incident Stress Management (CISM). *International Journal of Emergency Mental Health* **3**(1): 5–10, 2001.

Risk

Risk assessment – violence

Risk is the likelihood of behaviour that may be harmful or beneficial to oneself or to others. Risk assessment involves analysing potential outcomes of this behaviour; and risk management involves devising a care plan to minimize harmful behaviour and maximize beneficial behaviour.

Prevalence of violence in the UK

- There were 95,501 violent incidents in the NHS in 2002
- Mental health and learning disability settings had three times the national average of violent incidents
- A violent incident occurs every 3.5 days in London.

Consequences of violence

- Sickness from work
- Physical injury, sometimes serious
- Post-traumatic stress disorder (PTSD)
- A profound sense of alienation
- Persistent fear.

Demographic predictors of violence

- Previous history of violence to people or property
- History of misuse of substances or alcohol
- Previous expression of intent to harm others
- Evidence of rootlessness or social restlessness
- Previous dangerous or impulsive acts
- Previous use of weapons
- Denial of previous dangerous acts
- Verbal threats of violence.

Clinical predictors of violence

- Misuse of drugs or alcohol
- Drug effects (e.g. disinhibition)
- Delusions or hallucinations focused on a particular person
- Command hallucinations i.e. responding to voices commanding a certain act
- Preoccupation with violent fantasy
- Delusions of control
- Agitation, excitement, overt hostility, or suspicion
- Poor collaboration with suggested treatments
- Organic dysfunction e.g. forms of dementia.

Situational predictors of violence

- Extent of social support
- Immediate availability of potential weapon
- Relationship to victim
- Access to potential victim
- Staff setting limits on users
- Staff attitudes.

Patrick Callaghan Professor of Mental Health Nursing, University of Nottingham & Nottinghamshire Healthcare NHS Trust

Antecedents and warning signs

- Tense and angry facial expressions
- Increased or prolonged restlessness
- General over-arousal
- Increased volume of speech, erratic movements
- Prolonged eye contact
- Discontentment, refusal to communicate, withdrawal, fear, irritation
- Unclear thought processes, poor concentration
- Delusions or hallucinations with violent content
- Verbal threats or gestures
- Reporting anger or violent feelings
- Replicating previous behaviour that led to violence.

Risk assessment

Assessment should:
- Be regular and comprehensive
- Involve an assessment of staff attitudes, situations, organizational and environmental factors linked to violence
- Include a structured and sensitive interview with the user, to focus on triggers, early warning signs and other vulnerabilities
- Avoid negative assumptions based on ethnicity
- Involve a multidisciplinary approach
- Assess and record users preferences for managing violence.

Actuarial measures used in risk assessment

- Psychopathy checklist (PCL-R)
- Violence risk appraisal guide (VRAG)
- Historical/clinical/risk management 20 item scale (HCR-20)
- Dangerous Behaviour Rating Scale (DBRS).

Further reading

Moghan, S. Clinical Risk Management: A Clinical Tool and Practitioner Manual. The Sainsbury Centre for Mental Health: London, 2000.

National Institute of Health and Clinical Excellence. Violence: The Short Term management of disturbed/violent behaviour in psychiatric in-patient settings and emergency departments. Clinical Guideline 25. NICE: London, 2005.

Risk assessment – suicide

Risk is the likelihood of behaviour that may be harmful or beneficial to oneself or to others. Risk assessment involves analysing the potential outcomes of this behaviour; and risk management involves devising a care plan to minimize harmful behaviour and maximize beneficial behaviour.

Assessing suicide risk
- Risk factors
- History
- Information from relatives and carers
- Ideation/mental state
- Intent
- Planning
- Person's awareness of risk
- Benefits and harm from risk
- Formulation.

Predictors of suicide risk
- History of self-harm
- Depression
- Dual diagnosis
- Inpatient care
- Loss of contact with mental health services within one week of discharge
- Member of an ethnic minority
- Homelessness.

Risk factors of suicide

Higher risk	Lower risk
Males >65, males 15–30	Younger females
Separated, widowed, divorced	Married/stable relationship
Live alone, socially isolated	Good social network
Poor physical health	Good physical and mental health
Poor mental health	No previous episodes, no substance misuse, no family history
Substance misuse	
Previous episodes of self-harm	
Actual or attempted self-harm/ suicide by relative	
Loss of supports	
Hopelessness, despair, loss of interest	
Mild learning difficulty	

Patrick Callaghan, Professor of Mental Health Nursing, University of Nottingham & Nottinghamshire Healthcare NHS Trust

Aims of risk assessment

To establish:

- **If there is ongoing suicidal intent** such as a continuing wish to die, sense of hopelessness, or ambivalence about survival.
- **If there is evidence of mental illness** e.g. depressive illnesses or alcohol dependence.
- **If there are any non-mental health issues to address** e.g. emotional problems, family and/or relationship difficulties, school, employment, debt, or legal problems.

Assessment of needs

This should be comprehensive. It should include an evaluation of social, psychological and motivational factors specific to acts of self-harm, current suicidal intent, and an assessment of mental and social needs.

Assessment of risk

This should include:

- Identifying the main clinical and demographic features associated with risk of further self-harm.
- Identifying key psychological characteristics associated with risk e.g. depression, hopelessness, and continuing intent.

Further reading

National Institute of Health and Clinical Excellence. Self-Harm: The short-term physical and psychological management and secondary prevention of self-harm in primary and secondary care-Clinical Guideline 16. NICE: London, 2004.

Semple, D, Smyth, R, Burns, J, et al. Oxford Handbook of Psychiatry. Oxford University Press: Oxford, 2005.

Risk assessment – abuse

Risk is the likelihood of behaviour that may be harmful or beneficial to oneself or to others. Risk assessment involves analysing potential outcomes of this behaviour; and risk management involves devising a care plan to minimize harmful behaviour and maximize beneficial behaviour.

Types of abuse
- *Physical* – includes punching, pushing, hitting.
- *Sexual* – includes rape, sexual assault, sexual acts without consent or where consent could not be given.
- *Psychological* – includes emotional abuse, threats, humiliation.
- *Financial* – includes theft, fraud, exploitation.
- *Neglect* – includes ignoring needs, withholding the necessities of life.
- *Discrimination* – includes racism, sexism, ageism, harassment.
- *Institutional* – includes poor professional service, ill treatment.

Risk factors associated with abuse
For all types of abuse the risk factors are: unequal power, social isolation, and a vulnerable family history of violence and abuse.
Other risk factors are:
Physical abuse – long delays in reporting injuries, unexplained bruises, misuse of medication.
Sexual abuse – overly sexual conversations and behaviour.
Psychological abuse – ambivalence about carer, unexplained paranoia, passivity or resignation.
Financial abuse – unusual account activity, excessive gifts to carers.
Neglect – person left alone in unsafe environment, refusal of access to visitors or callers, violating privacy and dignity.
Rights violation – coercion, refusal of access to visitors or callers, lack of respect, lack of attention to personal hygiene.
Institutional – rigid routines, poor standards of cleanliness, 'batch' care.

Risk assessment
- Conduct assessment interview.
- Perform a mental state assessment.
- Take a history of abuse incidents.
- Assess specific indicators of abuse (see above).
- Assess for discrepancy between what is reported and what is observed.
- Assess for discrepancy between verbal and non-verbal cues.
- Assess coping potential and availability of social support.

Assessing the seriousness of abuse
- Vulnerability of the individual.
- Nature and extent of the abuse.
- Length of time of the abuse.
- Impact on the individual.

Patrick Callaghan, Professor of Mental Health Nursing, University of Nottingham & Nottinghamshire Healthcare NHS Trust

- Repeated or increasingly serious acts of abuse.
- Intent of person alleged responsible for the abuse.

Management of abuse

- Ensure safety of the victim.
- Discuss concerns with colleagues or multidisciplinary team.
- Make appropriate referrals to care management team, social services team, police/registration inspection unit.
- Consider what treatment or therapy is appropriate.
- Ensure modification in the way that services are provided.
- Support the individual through appropriate action he or she takes to seek justice or redress.
- Use stress management techniques.
- Encourage the vulnerable person to remain active and independent, maintaining social contacts.
- Work with significant others to discuss best forms of support or aftercare.

Further reading

Department of Health. Domestic Violence: A resources manual for health care professionals. DoH: London, 2000.

Oxleas Mental Health Trust. *A Guide to the assessment and management of risk.* Oxleas MH Trust: London, 2002: pp. 37–59.

Risk assessment – self-neglect

Risk is the likelihood of behaviour that may be harmful or beneficial to oneself or to others. Risk assessment involves analysing potential outcomes of this behaviour; and risk management involves devising a care plan to minimize harmful behaviour and maximize beneficial behaviour.

Risk factors to consider in assessment for self-neglect

- Hygiene
- Diet
- Physical health
- Medication
- Substance misuse
- Adequacy of clothing
- Capacity to self-care
- Capacity to seek help
- Adequacy of accommodation
- Household safety
- Basic household amenities
- Infestation
- Financial situation.

Risk factors linked to self-neglect

Higher risk	Lower risk
Female	Male
Living alone	Living with others
Mental illness; dementia, psychosis	Good health
Single, widowed, separated	Married/stable relationship
Substance misuse	No substance misuse
Poor housing	No loss of significant other
Loss of significant other	Good accommodation
Poor physical health	No cognitive or sensory impairments
Sensory and cognitive impairments	Living with competent carers
Unable to seek help	Able to seek help
Vulnerable to exploitation	

Risk assessment

- Take a history – awareness of illness/vulnerability, capacity to identify, understand, and manage risks, engagement with treatment or services, and pre-morbid personality.
- Discover the view of significant others – any expressions of concern.
- Assess ideation and mental state – capacity to make decisions and think about ways to manage risks, willingness to accept support, present state examination.

Patrick Callaghan, Professor of Mental Health Nursing, University of Nottingham & Nottinghamshire Healthcare NHS Trust

- Assess intent – the degree of intent to engage in a risky behaviour.
- Planning – assess whether the person has made any plans to engage in risky behaviour.
- Assess awareness of risk – the person's view of the problem.
- Assess the benefit versus the harm of risky behaviour.

Deciding on the nature and severity of the risk

1. How serious is the risk?
2. Is the risk specific or general?
3. How immediate is the risk?
4. How volatile is the risk?
5. Are circumstances likely to arise that will increase the risk?
6. What specific treatment and management plan can best reduce the risk?

Management

- The care programme approach (CPA 📖 Chapter 1) is important. Plan care with user and significant others.
- Identify antecedents of self-neglect behaviour (see above).
- Increased monitoring.
- Access to supported housing.
- Use of Section 117 if necessary.
- Environmental Health assessment and treatment of property if necessary.

Further reading

Johnson, J, Adams, J. Self-neglect in later life. *Health and Social Care in the Community* **4**(4): 226–33, 1996.

Oxleas Mental Health Trust. *A Guide to the assessment and management of risk.* Oxleas MH Trust: London, 2002: pp. 23–35.

Risk assessment – falls

Risk is the likelihood of behaviour that may be harmful or beneficial to oneself or to others. Risk assessment involves analysing potential outcomes of this behaviour; and risk management involves devising a care plan to minimize harmful behaviour and to maximize beneficial behaviour.

General areas to cover in assessment

- Risk factors
- History
- Physical health
- Environmental factors
- Information from relatives and carers
- Ideation/mental state
- Intent
- Planning
- Person's awareness of risk
- Benefits and harm of risk
- Formulation.

Risk assessment of falls

- Assess current symptoms
- Take a history of previous falls, noting in particular: **L**ocation, **A**ctivity, **T**ime, **T**rauma. Assess significant others' views
- Assess ideation and mental state – awareness of illness, vulnerability, capacity to make decisions
- Assess awareness of risk
- Consider the benefit and harm from risk
- Identification of falls history
- Assessment of gait, balance, mobility, and muscle weakness
- Assessment of osteoporosis risk
- Assessment of person's perceived functional ability, and fear of falling
- Assessment of visual impairment
- Assessment of cognitive impairment and neurological examination
- Assessment of urinary incontinence
- Assessment of home hazards
- Cardiovascular examination and review.

Multi-factorial management

- Strength and balance training
- Home hazard assessment and intervention
- Vision assessment and referral for treatment if necessary
- Medication review with modification/withdrawal
- Cardiac pacing
- Oral and written information to users and significant others about recommended measures to prevent further falls, and how to cope with a fall.

Patrick Callaghan, Professor of Mental Health Nursing, University of Nottingham & Nottinghamshire Healthcare NHS Trust

Rating scales for assessing falls risk
FRASE (Falls Risk Assessment for Elderly)
STRATIFY (St Thomas Risk Assessment Tool in Falling Elderly)

Risk factors of falls

Variable	Higher risk	Lower risk
Age	Older	Younger
Past history	Incidence of falls in past 12 months	No history of falls
Physical status	Medical problems especially circulatory	No/few medical problems
Environment	Hazardous	No hazards
Mental state	Sensory and cognitive impairment	No sensory or cognitive impairments
Medication	Combinations affecting balance	Combinations that do not affect balance
Mobility	Poor: gait/balance problems	No problems

Further reading
National Institute of Health and Clinical Excellence. Falls: the assessment and prevention of falls in older people, Guideline 21. NICE: London, 2004.
Oxleas Mental Health Trust. A Guide to the assessment and management of risk. Oxleas MH Trust: London, 2002: pp. 107–17.

Risk assessment – fire

Risk is the likelihood of behaviour that may be harmful or beneficial to oneself or to others. Risk assessment involves analysing potential outcomes of this behaviour; and risk management involves devising a care plan to minimize harmful behaviour and maximize beneficial behaviour.

Areas to cover in assessment

- Risk factors
- History
- Information from relatives and carers
- Ideation/mental state
- Intent
- Planning
- Person's awareness of risk
- Benefits and harm of risk
- Formulation.

Risk assessment

- Assess the person – do they exhibit risk factors? Do they exhibit safety awareness?
- Assess the environment – is there potential fuel for fires? Is there a fire alerting system? Is there a potential fire escape, and is the person able to use it?
- Other people – is there a potential risk to others?

Assessment of nature of previous fires

- *Timing* – how recent was the risk or behaviour?
- *Severity*
- *Frequency* – was it an isolated incident, or does it happen frequently?
- *Pattern* – is there a common pattern to the type of incident or the context in which it occurs?

Management of risk of fires

- Arrange further specialist assessment
- Admission to hospital if arson intent is present
- Make the person's environment safer
- Provide fire alerting devices
- Ensure supervision during procedures that may be risky, such as cooking, smoking, using appliances.

Patrick Callaghan, Professor of Mental Health Nursing, University of Nottingham & Nottinghamshire Healthcare NHS Trust

Risk factors – Fires

Variable	Higher risk	Lower risk
Past history of arson	Past history especially recent, younger age at first fire setting	No history
Past history of accidental fire setting	Past history especially recent	No history
Use of potential sources of fire	Poor safety awareness	Good safety awareness
	Smoker	Non-smoker
	Unsafe appliances	Safe appliances
	Unsafe behaviour, e.g. leaving pots unattended, leaving gas on, overloading electric circuits	Safe behaviour
Environment	Potential fuel for fire	Little potential fuel for fire
	No fire alerting system	Fire alerting system, e.g. working smoke alarm
	Electrical cords under furniture or carpeting	
Learning disability	Mild learning disability with poor social and communication skills	Severe learning disability

Further reading

Oxleas Mental Health Trust. *A Guide to the assessment and management of risk*. Oxleas MH Trust: London, 2002: pp. 119-230.

Common mental disorders

Anorexia nervosa

Anorexia nervosa is a condition where there is a marked distortion of body image, low weight, and weight loss behaviours. There is a mortality rate of 10–15% (two thirds due to physical complications and one third due to suicide).

Incidence

0.5% of adolescent and young women develop anorexia nervosa. There is a 1:10 ratio of males:females. There is equal distribution across social classes with mostly upper and middle class people seeking treatment.

Criteria

- Low body weight – 15% below expected BMI.
- Self induced weight loss – vomiting, purging, excessive exercise, use of appetite suppressants and laxatives.
- Body image distortion – dread of fatness, imposed low weight threshold.
- Endocrine disorders – involving the hypothalamus, pituitary, or adrenal glands.
- Amenorrhoea, reduced sexual interest or impotence, small body frame, altered thyroid function.
- Delayed puberty – if the onset is prior to puberty.

Aetiology

- Genetic – 6–10% of female siblings develop the condition.
- Life events – physical or sexual abuse *can be risk factors.*
- Psychodynamic –
  - Family relationships may be rigid, over protective, weak parental boundaries, lack of conflict resolution.
  - Individual – disturbed body image due to dietary problems in early life, parents' preoccupation with food, lack of sense of identity.
  - Analytical – regression to childhood, fixation on the oral stage, avoidance of problems in adolescence.

Mental health symptoms	Physical health symptoms	Common physical signs
Decreased concentration	General health concerns	Loss of muscle mass
Poor memory	Amenorrhoea	Dry skin
Irritability	Cold hands and feet	Brittle hair and nails
Depression	Weight loss	Anaemia
Low self-esteem	Constipation	Calluses on finger joints
Loss of appetite	Hair loss	Fine downy body hair
Reduced energy	Headaches	Eroded teeth enamel
Insomnia	Fainting or dizziness	Hypotension
Loss of libido	Lethargy	Bradycardia
Social withdrawal	Pale	Atrophy of the breasts
Obsessiveness with food		Swollen tender abdomen
Reduced decision-making		Loss of sensation in extremities

Prognosis

- If untreated, this condition carries one of the highest mortality rates for any mental health disorder.
- If treated, one third of patients make a full recovery, one third make a partial recovery, and one third have chronic problems.
- Most people are treated as an outpatient, with a combined approach including:
  - *Pharmacological* – antidepressants, medication to stimulate appetite.
  - *Psychological* – family therapy (may be effective if early onset). Individual therapy such as cognitive behavioural therapy (CBT) may improve long term outcomes.
  - *Education* – nutritional and self-help manuals
- Hospital admission should only be considered if there are serious medical problems. Compulsory admission may be required – feeding is regarded as treatment. Ethical issues have to be considered regarding a person's right to die, and their right to treatment.
- Poor prognostic factors include: chronic illness, late age of onset, bulimic features, anxiety when eating with others, excessive weight loss, poor childhood social adjustment, poor parental relationships, males.

📖 Working with a person with anorexia nervosa

Further reading

Duker, M, Slade, R. *Anorexia Nervosa and Bulimia.* Open University Press: Buckingham, 2002.
Eivors, A, Nesbitts, *Hunger for Understanding: a workbook for helping young people to understand and overcome anorexia nervosa.* John Wiley & Sons: 2005. Chichester UK.

Bulimia nervosa

Bulimia nervosa is a condition characterized by recurrent episodes of binge eating, combined with compensatory behaviours and overvalued ideas about ideal body shape and weight. Body weight may be normal, although there is often a past history of anorexia nervosa (30–50%).

Incidence

1–1.5% of women with onset during mid adolescence, and presentation in the early 20s.

Aetiology

Similar to anorexia nervosa. There is also evidence for associated personal or family history of affective disorder and/or substance misuse.

Criteria

- Persistent preoccupation with eating.
- Irresistible craving for food.
- Episodes of overeating (binging).
- Attempts to counter the fattening effects of food with self-induced vomiting, purgative abuse, periods of starvation, or use of appetite suppressants and laxatives.
- Morbid dread of fatness with imposed low weight threshold.

Physical signs

- May be similar to anorexia nervosa, but may be less severe
- Specific problems related to purging (laxative abuse)
  - Arrhythmias
  - Cardiac failure (sudden death)
  - Electrolyte disturbance due to laxatives or vomiting
  - Oesophageal erosion due to excessive vomiting
  - Oesophageal/gastric perforation
  - Gastric/duodenal ulcers
  - Pancreatitis
  - Constipation/steatorrhea
  - Dental erosions
  - Leucopenia/lymohytosis.

Treatment

- General principles:
  - Usually managed as an outpatient
  - Admission only for suicidality, physical problems, or pregnancy
  - Combined approaches improve outcome.
- Medication: there is evidence for high dose anti-depressants as long-term treatment.
- Psychotherapy:
  - Best evidence for CBT.
  - Interpersonal therapy is effective in the long-term, but acts less quickly.
  - Guided self-help is a useful first step, with education and support; often in a group setting.

Helen Waldock, Health and Social Care Advisory Service

Prognosis

Generally very good, unless there are issues of low self-esteem or severe personality disorder.

The SCOFF questions[1]

These questions are useful as a screening tool for eating disorders and can be used in any setting. A positive answer to two or more questions indicates that a further, more detailed history is indicated before considering treatment:

1. Do you make yourself sick because you feel uncomfortably full?
2. Do you worry that you have lost control over how much you eat?
3. Have you recently lost more than one stone in a three month period?
4. Do you believe yourself to be fat when others say you are too thin?
5. Would you say that food dominates your life?

📖 Working with a person with bulimia nervosa

Reference

1 Morgan, JF, Reid F, Lacey, JH. The SCOFF questionnaire: assessment of a new screening tool for eating disorders. *British Medical Journal* **319**: 1467–8, 1999.

Further reading

Duker, M, Slade, R. *Anorexia Nervosa and Bulimia*. Open University Press: Buckingham, 2002.
Semple, D, *Oxford Handbook of Psychiatry*. Oxford University Press: Oxford, 2005.

Schizophrenia

Schizophrenia is a highly variable disorder characterized by disordered perception, disordered thoughts (hallucinations and delusions), and withdrawal of the individuals interest from other people and the outside world.

Schizophrenia is a form of psychosis. Psychiatrists usually talk about 'schizophrenias' given the variability of this disorder. It typically develops in the late teens or early twenties, although males tend to have an earlier onset than females, and may develop more serious illness.

The symptoms of schizophrenia are divided into positive (new symptoms) and negative (loss of a previous function) symptoms.

Positive symptoms	Negative symptoms	Other symptoms
Delusions	Loss of motivation	Thought disorder
Hallucinations	Loss of social awareness	Agitation
	Flattened mood	Depression
	Poor abstract thinking	Poor sleep
		Cognitive impairment

The following symptoms have a special significance for diagnosis as they occur often in schizophrenia and more rarely in other disorders (sometimes referred to as first rank symptoms):

Symptoms	
Auditory hallucinations	Voices heard arguing
	Thought echo
	Running commentary on what the person is doing
Delusions or thought interference	Thought insertion
	Thought withdrawal
	Thought broadcasting
Delusions of control	Passivity of affect
	Passivity of impulse
	Passivity of volitions
	Somatic passivity
Delusional perceptions	A primary delusion of any context reported by the person as having arisen from a normal perception

Helen Waldock, Health and Social Care Advisory Service

Schizophrenia can be sub-classified on the basis of symptoms:

ICD-10	DSM-IV	Key symptoms
Paranoid schizophrenia	Paranoid type	Delusions and hallucinations
Hebephrenic schizophrenia	Disorganized type	Disorganized speech and behaviour(often silly/shallow) with flat or inappropriate manner
Catatonic schizophrenia	Catatonic type	Psychomotor disturbance such as mutism, posturing, rigidity, staring
Undifferentiated schizophrenia	Undifferentiated type	Meeting general criteria but no specific symptom subtype dominates
Post schizophrenia depression		Some residual symptoms but depressive picture dominates
Residual schizophrenia	Residual type	Previous positive symptoms less marked with prominent negative symptoms
Simple schizophrenia		No delusions or hallucinations, negative symptoms gradually arise without an acute episode

Epidemiology
- Prevalence: lifetime risk is between 7–13 per 1000 of the population.
- Mortality: suicide is the most common cause of premature death; accounting for 10–38% of all deaths.
- Genetic factors: account for 46% of identical twins, 40% both parents, 12–25% one parent, 12–15% sibling or non-identical twin, 6% grandparent, 0.5–1% no relative affected.
- Environmental factors: complications of pregnancy, delivery, and the neonatal period; delayed walking and neurodevelopmental difficulties; early social services contact and disturbed childhood behaviour, and winter births.

Prognosis
- Approximately 15–20% of first episodes will not occur again.
- Few people will remain in employment.
- 52% will be without psychotic symptoms in the last two years.
- 52% are without negative symptoms.
- 55% show good/fair social functioning.

Poor prognostic indicators include: poor pre-morbid adjustment, insidious onset, early onset, cognitive impairment, enlarged ventricles.
Good prognostic factors include: marked mood disturbance especially elation during initial presentation, family history of affective disorder, female, living in a developed country.

📖 Working with people with a perceptual disorder

Further reading
Mortensen, PB, Juel, K. Mortality and causes of death in first admitted schizophrenic patients. *British Journal of Psychiatry* **163**: 183–9, 1993.
Semple, D, Smyth R, Burns J, Darjee R, McIntosh A. *Oxford Handbook of Psychiatry*. Oxford University Press: Oxford, 2005.

Depression

In everyday language 'depression' refers to any downturn in mood; it may be relatively transitory and perhaps due to something trivial. Clinical depression is different. It is marked by symptoms that last two weeks or more, and are so severe that they interfere with daily living. It is not secondary to the use of drugs or alcohol.

Core symptoms of depression

- Depressed mood – present for most of the day, nearly every day, with little variation, and little responsiveness to environmental changes. There may be diurnal variation in mood – worse in the morning and improving as the day goes on.
- Anhedonia – diminished interest or pleasure in all, or almost all, activities most of the day, nearly every day (subjective account or observation by others).
- Weight change – loss of weight when not dieting, or a weight gain (of more than 5% of body weight within a month) associated with an increase or decrease in appetite.
- Disturbed sleep – insomnia with early morning wakening (2–3 hours sooner than usual) or hypersomnia, especially in atypical depression.
- Psychomotor agitation or retardation – observable by others, not just subjective feelings of restlessness or being slowed down.
- Fatigue or loss of energy.
- Feelings of worthlessness, or excessive inappropriate guilt (which may be delusional) – not just self-reproach or guilt about being ill.
- Reduced libido.
- Diminished ability to think or concentrate.
- Indecisiveness.
- Recurrent thought of death or suicide (not fear of dying), which may or may not have been acted upon.

Some of these symptoms are called 'somatic' or biological, such as anhedonia, loss of emotional reactivity, early morning wakening, and loss of appetite, weight, and libido.

Psychotic symptoms

- *Delusions* – poverty, personal inadequacy, guilt, assumed responsibility for world events, accidents or natural disasters.
- *Hallucinations* – auditory: defamatory or accusatory voices; olfactory: bad smells such as rotting food or faeces; visual: tormentors, demons, dead bodies.
- *Catatonic symptoms* – marked psychomotor retardation (depressive stupor).

Helen Waldock, Health and Social Care Advisory Service

Aetiology

Depression is likely to be caused by interplay of biological, psychological, and social factors:

- *Genetic factors* – individual's sensitivity to life stressors.
- *Personality factors* – enduring traits with a biological basis such as a positive attitude, or being 'laid back' which mediates the response to external stimuli or events.
- *Psychological factors* – the disruption of normal social, marital, parental or familial relationships is correlated with high rates of depression.
- *Gender* – there is an increased prevalence in women, possibly due to restricted social and occupational roles, ruminative response styles and endocrine factors, or it may be that women are more likely to admit to these types of problems.
- *Social factors* – lower levels of income, employment, and education are predisposing factors; the stress associated with these problems leads to depression.
- *Social* isolation – a key risk factor especially for those who already have an established mental health problem.

Prognosis

Suicide rates vary, up to 13% for severe depression, higher for those who have required hospital admission.

Good outcome: acute onset, endogenous (from within, not related to an external event), and young.

Poor outcome: slow onset, neurotic features, elderly, residual symptoms. Low confidence, alcohol or drug misuse, personality disorders, physical illness, or lack of social support.

📖 Working with people with a mood disorder

Further reading

National Institute for Mental Health website: www.nimh.nih.gov.uk

Semple, D, Smyth R, Burns J, Darjee R, McIntosh A. *Oxford Handbook of Psychiatry.* Oxford University Press: Oxford, 2005.

Substance misuse

Substance misuse refers to the harmful use of any substance, such as alcohol, a street drug, or the misuse of a prescribed drug.

Features of substance misuse disorder

- **Acute intoxication** – the pattern of reversible physical and mental abnormalities caused by the direct effect of the substance such as disinhibition, ataxia, euphoria, and visual and sensory distortion.
- **At risk use** – a pattern of substance use where the person is at increased risk of harming their physical or mental health. This can be normal consumption or harmful use. It does not depend on the amounts taken, but on the situations and associated behaviors e.g. alcohol and driving.
- **Harmful use** – the continuation of substance misuse despite evidence of damage to the person's mental health, social, occupational, or familial well-being. Damage is denied or minimized.
- **Dependence** – includes both physical and psychological dependence.
- **Withdrawal** – physical dependence where abstinence leads to features of withdrawal. Different substances produce different symptoms; often the opposite of the acute effects of the substance. Clinically significant withdrawals are recognized in alcohol, opiates, benzodiazepines, amphetamines, and cocaine.
- **Complicated withdrawal** – development of seizures, delirium or psychotic features.
- **Substance induced psychotic disorder** – hallucinations and/or delusions occurring as a direct result of substance neurotoxicity. Features may occur during intoxication or withdrawal states. It is differentiated from primary psychotic illness by the symptoms being non-typical e.g. late first presentation, prominence of non-auditory hallucinations.
- **Cognitive impairment syndromes** – reversible cognitive deficits occur during intoxication, and persist in chronic misuse amounting to dementia. Most common in alcohol, volatile chemicals, benzodiazepines, and possibly cannabis.
- **Residual disorders** – continuing symptoms exist despite discontinuing the substance.
- **Exacerbation of pre-existing disorder** – all other psychiatric illnesses, especially anxiety, panic disorders, mood disorders, and psychotic disorders may be associated with co-morbid substance misuse. This results in an exacerbation of the patient's symptoms and a decline in the effectiveness of treatment.

The dependence syndrome

The dependence syndrome describes the features of substance dependence:

- Primacy of drug seeking behavior – it is the most important thing in the person's life, taking priority over all activities and interests.
- Narrowing the drug taking repertoire – the person takes a single substance in preference to all others.

Helen Waldock, Health and Social Care Advisory Service

- Increased tolerance to the effects of the drug – increased amounts are needed to achieve the same effect, the person explores other routes such as intravenous.
- Loss of control of consumption – there is an inability to restrict further consumption.
- Signs of withdrawal on attempted abstinence.
- Drug taking to avoid withdrawal symptoms.
- Continued drug use despite negative consequences, such as marital break up, prison sentence, loss of job.
- Rapid reinstatement of previous pattern of drug use after abstinence.

📖 Working with the person with substance misuse
📖 Principles of working with service users with substance misuse problems

Further reading

Edwards, G, Gross, MM. Alcohol dependence: provisional description of a clinical syndrome. *British Medical Journal* **1**: 1058-61, 1976.
Semple, D, Smyth R, Burns J, Darjee R, McIntosh A. *Oxford Handbook of Psychiatry*. Oxford University Press: Oxford, 2005.

Personality disorder

The term personality disorder is one of the most contentious diagnoses in psychiatry; it is often used as a pejorative label for patients who are unpopular. Diagnostic reliability is poor despite clear diagnostic criteria.

Personality disorders begin in childhood or adolescence and continue into adulthood. They are persistent pervasive disorders of inner experience and behaviour that cause distress or significant impairment of social functioning.

A personality disorder can show itself in problems of:
- Cognition – ways of perceiving and thinking about oneself and others.
- Affect – the range, intensity, and appropriateness of emotional response.
- Behaviour – interpersonal, occupational, and social functioning.

There are two schools of thought in the mental health professions for and against diagnosing personality disorder (PD). This has been superseded by the publication of the document Personality Disorder: no longer a diagnosis of exclusion.[2]

For the diagnosis	Against the diagnosis
Those with PD suffer with the symptoms of their condition	Personality is by definition unchangeable
There is a high rate of suicide, premature death and other mental illness	There is no evidence that psychiatry can do anything
Some treatment approaches are effective	Those with PD are disruptive and impinge negatively on staff and other patients
Services are traditional and do not provide the type of approach required	Those with PD are not ill and are responsible for their behaviour
	They are basically a social problem

Aetiology

There is no single theory for the causes of personality disorder. The following may be relevant:
- Genetics – there is some evidence of a link between affective disorder and borderline personality disorder; delusional disorder and paranoid personality disorder.
- Childhood development – a difficult infant temperament may proceed to conduct disorder in childhood and personality disorder in adulthood; ADHD and family pathology are possible risk factors for antisocial personality disorder, sexual abuse may predispose for borderline personality disorder.
- Psychodynamic theories – Freudian explanations of arrested development at oral, anal, and genital stages leading to narcissistic and borderline personality with primitive defence mechanisms and projective identification (including splitting).

Helen Waldock, Health and Social Care Advisory Service

- Cognitive behaviour theories – maladaptive core beliefs derived from an interaction between childhood experience and pre-programmed patterns of behaviour.
- Cognitive analytical model – experience a range of partially dissociated self states, in response to unmanageable external threats.
- Dialectical behaviour model – innate temperamental vulnerabilities interact with dysfunctional invalidating environments leading to problems with emotional regulation.

Classification of personality disorder

Personality disorder	Description
Paranoid	Sensitive, suspicious, preoccupied with conspiratorial explanations, self-referential, distrust of others
Schizoid	Emotionally cold, detached, lack of interest in others, excessive introspection and fantasy
Schizotypal	Interpersonal discomfort with peculiar ideas, perceptions, appearance, and behaviours
Antisocial	Callous lack of concern for others, irresponsibility, irritability, aggression, inability to maintain enduring relationships, disregard and violation of others' rights, evidence of childhood conduct disorder
Emotionally unstable	Inability to control anger or pain, with unpredictable affect and behaviour
Borderline	Unclear identity, intense and unstable relationships, unpredictable affect, frequent threats and acts of self-harm, impulsivity
Histrionic	Self-dramatization, shallow affect, egocentricity, craving attention and excitement, manipulative behaviour
Narcissistic	Grandiosity, lack of empathy, need for admiration
Avoidant	Tension, self-consciousness, fear of negative evaluation by others, timid and insecure
Obsessive-compulsive	Doubt, indecisiveness, caution, pedantry, rigidity, perfectionism, preoccupation with orderliness and control
Dependent	Clinging, submissive, excess need for care, feels helpless when not in a relationship

📖 Working with people with a personality disorder (PD)

Reference

2 Department of Health. Personality Disorder: no longer a diagnosis of exclusion. DoH: London, 2003.

Further reading

Linehan, M. *Cognitive Behaviour Treatment of Borderline Personality Disorder*. The Guilford Press: New York, 1993.
Sharpe, R. *A fractured mind: my life with multiple personality*. Souvenir Press Ltd: 2006. London.

Bipolar affective disorder

People with bipolar affective disorder can experience recurrent attacks of depression and mania or hypomania. It is commonly called manic depression, and is more common in women, with the average age of onset at around 21 years. Children of a parent with bipolar disorder have a 50% chance of developing a mental illness. There is no significant racial difference.

The course of the illness is extremely variable. The onset can be hypomanic, manic, mixed, or depressive; and this may be followed by five or more years without a further episode. The length of time between episodes may then begin to diminish. People with hypomania share the same symptoms as mania, but to a lesser degree, and the condition may not significantly disrupt work or lead to social rejection.

Core features of mania
- Elevated mood, usually out of keeping with circumstances.
- Increased energy, which may manifest as:
  - Over activity.
  - Pressured speech (flight of ideas).
  - Racing thoughts.
  - Reduced need for sleep.
- Increased self-esteem, evident as:
  - Over optimistic ideation.
  - Grandiosity.
  - Reduced social inhibitions.
  - Over familiarity (may be over amorous).
  - Facetiousness.
- Reduced attention span or increased distractibility.
- Tendency to engage in risk behaviour that could have serious consequences:
  - Preoccupation with extravagant impractical schemes.
  - Spending recklessly.
  - Inappropriate sexual encounters.
- Other behavioural manifestations:
  - Excitement.
  - Irritability.
  - Aggressiveness or suspiciousness.
- Disruption of work, usual social activities, and family life.

Psychotic symptoms
In severe mania, psychotic symptoms may develop:
- Grandiose ideas may become delusional with special powers or religious content.
- Suspiciousness may develop into well-formed persecutory delusions.
- Pressured speech may become so great that clear associations are lost and speech becomes incomprehensible.
- Irritability and aggression may lead to violent behaviour.

Helen Waldock, Health and Social Care Advisory Service

- Preoccupation with thoughts and schemes may lead to self-neglect to the point of not eating or drinking and living in dishevelled circumstances.
- Catatonic behaviour, also termed manic stupor.
- Total loss of insight and connection to the outside world.

Prognosis

Morbidity and mortality rates are high in terms of lost work, productivity, and effects on marriage and the family. 25–50% of people with bipolar affective disorder attempt suicide and 10% do kill themselves.

Poor prognosis is associated with, poor employment history, alcohol abuse, psychotic features, depression inbetween episodes of mania, being male, and not complying with medication.

Good prognosis is associated with manic episodes of short duration, later age at onset, few thoughts of suicide or symptoms of psychosis, good treatment response, and compliance.

Further reading

Fink, C, Kraynak, J. *Bipolar Disorder for Dummies*. John Wiley & Sons Ltd: 2005. New York.
Miklowitz, DJ. *The Bipolar Disorder Survival Guide: What you and your family need to know*. The Guilford Press: New York, 2002.
Semple, D. Smyth R, Burns J, Darjee R, McIntosh A. *Oxford Handbook of Psychiatry*. Oxford University Press: Oxford, 2005.

Obsessive-compulsive disorder (OCD)

Definition

The essential feature of this disorder is recurrent obsessional thoughts or compulsive acts. Obsessional thoughts are ideas, images, or impulses that enter a person's mind again and again. They are distressing because they are intrusive and irrational, and they may be violent or obscene. People can usually recognize their thoughts and compulsions as unreasonable and excessive; and often try unsuccessfully to resist them.

The average age of onset of OCD is around 20 years; it is prevalent in the population at 0.5–2% with an equal male:female distribution. The course of the condition is variable and more likely to be chronic in the absence of significant depressive symptoms.

Core features of OCD

- The obsessions or compulsions must be recognized as the person's own thoughts or impulses, even though they may be involuntary or repugnant.
- There must be at least one thought or act that is still resisted successfully, even though others may be present which the sufferer no longer resists.
- Carrying out the compulsion must not in itself be pleasurable (simple relief of tension or anxiety is not regarded as pleasure in this sense).
- The thoughts, images, or impulses must be intrusive and unpleasantly repetitive.

Categories/types of OCD

- Checking – 63%
- Washing – 50%
- Contamination – 45%
- Doubting – 42%
- Bodily fears – 36%
- Counting – 36%
- Insistence on symmetry – 31%
- Aggressive thoughts – 28%

Compulsions

Compulsive acts or rituals are stereotyped behaviours that are repeated again and again. They are not inherently enjoyable, nor do they result in the completion of an inherently useful task. Repeated attempts are made to resist the behaviour, although in very long-standing cases, resistance may be minimal. Autonomic anxiety symptoms are often present, but distressing feelings of internal or psychic tension without obvious autonomic arousal are also common.

Helen Waldock, Health and Social Care Advisory Service

Depression

There is a close relationship between compulsions and obsessional symptoms, particularly obsessional thoughts, and depression. People with obsessive-compulsive disorder often have depressive symptoms, and those suffering from recurrent depressive disorder may develop obsessional thoughts during their episodes of depression. In either situation, increases or decreases in the severity of the depressive symptoms are generally accompanied by parallel changes in the severity of the obsessional symptoms.

Prognosis

- 20–40% significantly improve, 40–50% show a moderate improvement.
- 20–40 have chronic or worsening symptoms.
- Relapse rates are high for stopping medication.

Poor prognosis – giving in to compulsions, longer duration, early onset, bizarre compulsions, symmetry, co-morbid depression, personality disorder.

Better prognosis – good pre-morbid social and occupational adjustment, a precipitating event, episodic symptoms.

Further reading

Deane, R. *Washing my life away: surviving obsessive compulsive disorder.* Jessica Kingsley Publishing: 2005. London .UK.

Semple, D, Smyth R, Burns J, Darjee R, McIntosh A. *Oxford Handbook of Psychiatry.* Oxford University Press: Oxford, 2005.

Swinson, RP. *Obsessive Compulsive Disorder: theory, research and treatment.* The Guilford Press: New York, 2001.

Anxiety

Definition

Anxiety is a normal and adaptive response to stress and danger. It is damaging if it is prolonged, severe, or out of keeping with the real threat of the external situation. Moderate amounts of anxiety can optimize performance, for example being nervous before a test or exam may help you perform better. The sensations of anxiety are related to autonomic arousal and cognitive appraisal of threat, which were adaptive primitive survival mechanisms. This is referred to as the 'fight or flight' instinct.

Anxiety has two components:

- Psychic anxiety – where there is subjective tension, increased arousal, and fearful apprehension.
- Somatic anxiety – bodily sensations such as palpitations, sweating, dyspnoea (shortness of breath), pallor, or abdominal discomfort.

Symptoms of anxiety

General symptoms of anxiety and tension – hot flushes or cold chills, numbness or tingling sensations, muscle tension, aches and pains, restlessness or an inability to relax, feeling keyed-up, on edge, or mentally tense, a sensation of a lump in the throat, or difficulty swallowing.

Physical symptoms – breathing difficulties, dry mouth, palpitations, choking sensation, chest pain or discomfort, tachycardia, sweating, trembling, nausea, and abdominal distress.

Mental state symptoms – feeling dizzy, unsteady, faint or light-headed, fear of losing control, 'going crazy', passing out, or dying.

Other symptoms – exaggerated response to minor surprises or being startled, concentration difficulties, mind going blank due to worry or anxiety, persistent irritability, difficulty getting to sleep due to worry.

Anxiety disorders

Generalized anxiety disorder (GAD)

Excessive worry, (free-floating and persistent), feelings of apprehension about everyday events or problems, with symptoms of muscle and psychic tension, causing significant distress and functional impairment.

Acute stress reaction

A transient disorder that may last for hours or days, and that may occur as an immediate (within one hour) response to exceptional circumstances e.g. after a major accident, assault, warfare, or rape. The stressor usually involves a severe threat to the security or physical integrity of the individual or a loved one.

Acute stress disorder

This overlaps with the acute stress reaction, with an emphasis on the symptoms of dissociation and hyper-arousal. Onset is usually within four weeks of an event, with symptoms lasting up to four weeks, after which post-traumatic stress disorder (PTSD) has to be considered.

Helen Waldock, Health and Social Care Advisory Service

Panic attack

A period of intense fear, that develops rapidly and reaches a peak of intensity at around 10 minutes (it does not generally last longer than 20–30 minutes) a panic attack may be spontaneous or situational, and can occur during sleep.

Panic disorder

This is diagnosed when a person has recurrent panic attacks that are not secondary to substance misuse, a medical condition, or another mental health problem.

📖 Working with people with an anxiety disorder

Further reading

Semple, D, Smyth R, Burns J, Darjee R, McIntosh A. *Oxford Handbook of Psychiatry*. Oxford University Press: Oxford, 2005.

Sharpe, R. *Self-Help for your Anxiety*. Souvenir Press: London, UK. 1997.

Phobias

Definition

Phobias are caused by fear of particular stimuli, events, or situations; the fear arouses symptoms of anxiety and the situations or sSstimuli are therefore associated with avoidance. The concept of biological prepared-ness is that some fears e.g. snakes, fire, heights, had an evolutionary advantage.

Signs

• Somatic physical symptoms such as blushing, trembling, or dry mouth when exposed to the object/situation (anxiety reactions such as: sweating, trembling, nausea, rapid heartbeat are common).
• Excessive fear (recognized as excessive by the individual) of humilia-tion, embarrassment, or others noticing how anxious they are.
• Individuals are characteristically critical and of perfectionist personality.
• Difficulty in maintaining social or sexual relationships, educational problems, difficulties in interactions with others or problems at work, caused by avoidance.
• Thoughts of suicide are relatively common.

Specific phobias

People with specific phobias experience excessive and unreasonable psychological or autonomic symptoms of severe anxiety and panic in the presence or anticipated presence of a specific feared object or situation, which leads to avoidance.

Phobias may begin in childhood, and are often brought on by a trau-matic event; being bitten by a dog, for example, may bring about a fear of dogs. Phobias that begin in childhood may disappear as the person grows older. There are five common categories of phobia:

• Animals e.g. hair, fur, skin (chaetophobia, trichophobia, doraphobia).
• Aspects of the natural environment e.g. forest at night (nyctohylo-phobia).
• Blood, injury, or injection (trypanophobia).
• Specific situations e.g. dentist, hospital (dentophobia, nosocome-phobia).

Other common phobias are choking and deep water (anginaphobia, bathophobia).

Social phobia

A social phobia is experienced as symptoms of incapacitating anxiety, which are not secondary to delusional or obsessive thoughts. These are restricted to particular social situations, leading to a desire for escape or avoidance (which may reinforce a strongly held belief of social inade-quacy). The onset of this phobia is usually mid to late adolescence.

Agoraphobia

Sometimes coincides with panic disorder. Agoraphobia is characterized by a fear of having a panic attack in a place from which it is difficult to escape. Many people with agoraphobia refuse to leave their homes, often for years at a time. Others develop a fixed route, or territory, from which they cannot deviate, such as the route between home and work. It becomes impossible to travel beyond what they consider to be their safety zone without suffering severe anxiety.

Claustrophobia

One of the most common phobias is claustrophobia, or the fear of enclosed spaces. A person who has claustrophobia may panic when inside a lift, an aeroplane, a crowded room, or other confined area. For a person with severe claustrophobia, a closed door may trigger feelings of panic.

Common claustrophobic behaviour:

- *Inside a room* – automatically checking for the exits, standing near the exits, or feeling alarmed when all doors are closed.
- *Inside a vehicle* – avoiding public transport or times when traffic is known to be heavy.
- *Inside a building* – preferring to take the stairs rather than the lift.
- *At a party* – standing near the door in a crowded room, even if the room is large and spacious.

Further reading

Beck, A, Emery, G. Anxiety Disorders and Phobias: a cognitive perspective. Basic Books: New York, 1990.
Website: www.jillschmitt.co.uk.

Sexual disorders – female

The primary characteristic of female sexual disorder is impairment in normal sexual functioning. This can refer to an inability to reach an orgasm, painful sexual intercourse, strong feelings of repulsion towards sexual activity, or an exaggerated sexual response cycle or sexual interest. For a sexual dysfunction diagnosis to be made the symptoms must be hindering the person's everyday functioning and any possible medical cause must be ruled out.

Female orgasmic disorder

Aetiology

Failure to achieve an orgasm for women is related to intimacy issues, feelings of fear and anxiety, and a sense of not being safe within the intimate relationship or relationships in general.

Symptoms

A delay of orgasm following normal excitement and sexual activity. Due to the widely varied sexual response in women, it must be judged by a clinician to be significant, taking into account the person's age and situation. For this diagnosis, the condition must be persistent or occur frequently and cause significant distress. Substance abuse must be ruled out.

Treatment

Typical treatment would involve discovering and resolving underlying conflicts or life difficulties through counselling or psychotherapy.

Prognosis

Very good. Especially if the underlying issues are addressed and worked through.

Female sexual arousal disorder

Aetiology

There is some evidence suggesting that relationship issues and/or sexual trauma in childhood may play a role in the development of this disorder.

Symptoms

An inability to attain or maintain, until sexual activity is complete, adequate lubrication in response to sexual excitement. For this diagnosis, the condition must result in significant distress and not be better accounted for by another disorder or the misuse of a substance such as estrogen depletion.

Treatment

Typical treatment would involve discovering and resolving underlying conflict or life difficulties e.g. with help of a therapist.

Prognosis

Varies, but increases with the ability to gain insight into and work through relationship issues or issues stemming from childhood which are playing a role in this disorder.

Helen Waldock Health and Social Care Advisory Service

Vaginismus

Aetiology
There is a relationship between this disorder and the victims of rape, sexual abuse, strict religious upbringing, and issues of control.

Symptoms
Recurrent or persistent involuntary spasms of the vaginal muscles that interfere with sexual intercourse. For this diagnosis to be made, it must cause significant distress, and other medical conditions or disorders must be ruled out.

Treatment
Psychological treatment that involves working through underlying issues; other treatments can involve progressively larger dilators, and therapy to help relax muscles which prevent intercourse.

Prognosis
Good.

📖 Assessing and managing the side effects of medication
📖 Sexuality and Mental Health-a research study
📖 Sexuality (sexual orientation) and mental health

Further reading
Website: www.allpsych.com
Icon Health Publications. *Female Sexual Dysfunction: A medical dictionary, bibliography and anno-tated research guide to internet references.* Icon Health San Diego: 2004.

Sexual disorders – male

Male orgasmic disorder

Aetiology

Male orgasmic disorder is often thought of as beginning in adolescence or early adulthood especially if sexual intimacy becomes linked to a negative life event or aspect. A medical cause must always be ruled out first.

Symptoms

The delay or absence of orgasm, following normal excitement and sexual activity. Due to the widely varied sexual response in men, it must be judged by a clinician to be significant, taking into account the person's age and situation. For a diagnosis to be made, the condition must be persistent or occur frequently and cause significant distress. The effect of substance abuse must also be ruled out.

Treatment

Once a medical cause is ruled out, working through the underlying issues can be very helpful. If the underlying issues are not significant, some therapists also use behavioural techniques such as sensate focus, which is a more direct approach.

Prognosis

Very good.

Male erectile disorder (impotence)

Aetiology

Previously referred to as impotence, any medical causes of this disorder must be ruled out first. Short of any physiological cause, male erectile disorder is typically a result of 'performance anxiety' or fears of not being able to achieve or maintain an erection.

Symptoms

The recurring inability to achieve or maintain an erection until sexual activity is complete. For this diagnosis to be made there must be significant distress for the individual, other disorders such as drug abuse or a physical problem must be ruled out.

Treatment

The most commonly used treatment for non-medical related impotence is 'sensate focus' through a qualified sex therapist or counselor. This involves a gradual progression of sexual intimacy, typically over the course of several weeks, eventually leading to penetration and orgasm.

Prognosis

Very good.

Helen Waldock, Health and Social Care Advisory Service

Premature ejaculation

Aetiology

Any medical causes must be ruled out first. Relationship stress, a new relationship, anxiety, or issues related to control and intimacy can all play a role in the development of this disorder.

Symptoms

Ejaculation with minimal sexual stimulation, before or shortly after penetration and before the person wishes it. For this diagnosis to be made the condition must be persistent or occur frequently and cause significant distress. The effect of substance use must also be ruled out.

Treatment

Relaxation training, education, and working through underlying issues are all treatment options. If the relationship is new, the difficulties will often resolve as the relationship matures.

Prognosis

Good.

📖 Assessing and managing the side effects of medication
📖 Sexuality and Mental Health-a research study
📖 Sexuality (sexual orientation) and mental health

Further reading

Website: www.allpsych.com
Icon Health Publications. *Male Sexual Dysfunction: A medical dictionary, bibliography and annotated research guide to internet references.* Icon Health, San Diego: 2004.

Sexual disorders – male and female

Gender identity disorder

Aetiology
Theories suggest that childhood issues may play a role in this disorder; for example, the early parent-child relationship, and the child's identification with the parent of the same gender.

Symptoms
A strong and persistent identification with the opposite gender. The person feels a sense of discomfort in their own gender and may feel they were 'born the wrong sex'. This disorder has been confused with cross-dressing or transvestic fetishism, but these are all separate conditions. Depression, anxiety, relationship difficulties, and personality disorders may also be present with gender identity disorder. Homosexuality is present in a majority of cases.

Treatment
Psychological treatment is likely to be long-term, with small gains made on underlying issues as treatment progresses. Gender reassignment is suitable for a minority of sufferers.

Prognosis
Mixed. The goals of treatment are not as clear as in other disorders, as same-sex identification may be very difficult to achieve. More achievable goals may include an acceptance of the assigned gender and resolution of other difficulties such as depression or anxiety.

Hypoactive sexual desire disorder

Aetiology
Some evidence suggests that relationship issues and/or sexual trauma in childhood may play a role in the development of this disorder. Life stressors or other interpersonal difficulties may also contribute.

Symptoms
Diagnosis must be made by a clinician taking into account the individual's age and life circumstances. The lack of desire experienced must result in significant distress for the individual and another disorder or physical problem must be ruled out.

Treatment
Typical treatment would involve discovering and resolving any underlying conflict or life difficulties *through counselling or therapy*.

Prognosis
The course of this disorder can be consistent or periodic, and can therefore resurface after a period of remission if relationship issues or life stressors re-emerge.

Helen Waldock, Health and Social Care Advisory Service

Sexual aversion disorder

Aetiology

Some evidence suggests that relationship issues and/or sexual trauma in childhood may play a role in the development of this disorder.

Symptoms

A persistent or recurring aversion to, or an avoidance of sexual activity. When presented with a sexual opportunity, the person may experience panic attacks or extreme anxiety. This aversion must result in significant distress for the individual; other disorders or physical problems must be ruled out.

Treatment

Typical treatment would involve discovering and resolving underlying conflict or life difficulties *through counseling or therapy*.

Prognosis

Increases with the ability to gain insight and work through relationship issues, or issues stemming from childhood which are playing a role in this disorder.

📖 Assessing and managing the side effects of medication
📖 Sexuality and Mental Health-a research study
📖 Sexuality (sexual orientation) and mental health

Further reading

Website: www.allpsych.com
Plaut M, Graziottin A, Heahon P.W. Fast Facts: Sexeual Dysfunction 2004. Oxford Health Press, Oxford UK.

Somatoform disorders

Somatoform disorders are a group of disorders characterized by physical symptoms suggesting a medical condition. They are classified as psychiatric conditions because the physical symptoms present cannot be fully explained by a medical disorder, substance use, or another mental disorder.

Body dysmorphic disorder

- A preoccupation with an imagined defect of appearance. If a slight physical anomaly is present, the person is excessively concerned.
- This preoccupation with appearance causes clinically significant distress, or impairment in social, occupational, or other important areas of functioning.
- The preoccupation is not caused by another disorder (e.g. dissatisfaction with body shape and size in anorexia nervosa).

Conversion disorder

- One or more symptoms or deficits affecting voluntary motor or sensory function that suggest a neurological or other general medical condition.
- Psychological factors are judged to be associated with the symptom or deficit, because its appearance is preceded by conflicts or other stressors.
- The symptom or deficit is not intentionally produced or feigned (as in factitious disorder or malingering).
- The symptom or deficit cannot be fully explained (after appropriate investigation) by a general medical condition, as a culturally sanctioned behaviour or experience, or by the direct effects of a substance misuse.
- The symptom or deficit causes clinically significant distress or impairment in social, occupational, or other important areas of functioning; or warrants medical intervention.
- The symptom or deficit is not limited to pain or sexual dysfunction, it does not occur exclusively during the course of somatization disorder (see opposite) and cannot be accounted for by another mental disorder.

Hypochondriasis

- Preoccupation with the fear of having, or the idea that one has, a serious disease, based on a misinterpretation of bodily symptoms.
- A preoccupation that persists despite appropriate medical evaluation and reassurance.
- A preoccupation that causes clinically significant distress or impairment in social, occupational, or other important areas of functioning.
- The duration of the disturbance is at least six months.
- The preoccupation is not better accounted for by generalized anxiety.

Helen Waldock, Health and Social Care Advisory Service

Somatization disorder

A history of many physical complaints – beginning before the age of 30 years – that occur over a period of several years and result in treatment being sought, or in significant impairment in social, occupational, or other important areas of functioning.

Each of the following criteria must be met, with individual symptoms occurring at any time during the course of the disturbance:

- Four pain symptoms – a history of pain related to at least four different sites or functions (e.g. head, abdomen, back, joints, extremities, chest, rectum, during menstruation, during sexual intercourse, or during urination).
- Two gastrointestinal symptoms – a history of at least two gastrointestinal symptoms other than pain (e.g. nausea, bloating, vomiting – other than during pregnancy, diarrhoea, or intolerance to several different foods).
- One sexual symptom – a history of at least one sexual or reproductive symptom other than pain (e.g. sexual indifference, erectile or ejaculatory dysfunction, irregular menses, excessive menstrual bleeding, vomiting throughout pregnancy).
- One pseudoneurological symptom – a history of at least one symptom or deficit suggesting a neurological condition not limited to pain (conversion symptoms such as impaired coordination or balance, paralysis or localized weakness, difficulty swallowing or loss of consciousness other than fainting).

📖 Working with specific physical and psychosomatic disorders

Further reading

Website: www.behavenet.com

Philips, KA. *Somatoform and Factitious Disorders*. American Psychiatric Pub Inc, 2001. Arlington, USA.

Neuropsychiatric disorders

Neuropsychiatry is at the interface of psychiatry and neurology. It is a specialist medical discipline, involving the behavioural or psychological difficulties associated with known or suspected neurological conditions. Technically, neuropsychiatry concentrates on abnormalities in those areas of higher brain function, such as the cerebral cortex and the limbic system.

Epilepsy

Epilepsy is a chronic neurological condition characterized by recurrent unprovoked seizures; it is often referred to as a seizure disorder. It is commonly controlled with medication, although surgical methods are used as well.

Seizures can be sub-classified into a number of categories, depending on their behavioural effects:

Absence seizures

These are sometimes called 'petit mal' seizures, and involve an interruption to consciousness, where the person affected seems to become vacant and unresponsive for a short period of time (usually up to 30 seconds). Slight muscle twitching may occur.

Tonic-clonic seizures

These are sometimes called 'grand mal' seizures. They involve an initial contraction of the muscles ('tonic' phase), which may result in tongue biting, urinary incontinence and the absence of breathing. This is followed by rhythmic muscle contractions ('clonic' phase). The colloquial term 'epileptic fit' refers to this type of seizure.

Myoclonic seizures

These involve sporadic muscle contraction and can result in jerky movements of muscles or muscle groups.

Atonic seizures

These involve the loss of muscle tone, causing the person to fall to the ground. They are sometimes called 'drop attacks,' but must be distinguished from similar looking attacks that may occur in narcolepsy or cataplexy.

Status epilepticus

This refers to continuous seizure activity with no recovery between successive tonic-clonic seizures. This is a life-threatening condition and if it is suspected, emergency medical assistance should be called immediately. A tonic-clonic seizure lasting longer than 5 minutes (or two minutes longer than an individual's usual seizures) is usually considered grounds for calling the emergency services.

Helen Waldock, Health and Social Care Advisory Service

Attention-deficit hyperactivity disorder (ADHD)

ADHD is one of the most commonly diagnosed mental disorders among children. It may be diagnosed in adults, if symptoms were present – even if undiagnosed – in childhood. Current theory holds that approximately 30% of children diagnosed with ADHD retain the disorder as adults. In adults, it is often referred to as adult attention-deficit disorder (AADD).

Tourette's syndrome

Tourette's syndrome is a neurological, or neurochemical disorder characterized by tics. These may be involuntary, rapid, sudden movements or vocalizations that occur repeatedly in the same way. The onset is usually before the age of 18.

Tics can be almost any short vocal sound, with the most common tics resembling throat clearing, short coughs, grunts, or moans. Motor tics can be of endless variety and may include hand-clapping, banging the knuckles together, and contorted facial grimacing.

Vocal tics may fall into various categories:
- *Echolalia* (the urge to repeat words spoken by someone else after being heard by the person with the disorder).
- *Palilalia* (the urge to repeat one's own previously spoken words).
- *Lexilalia* (the urge to repeat words after reading them).
- *Coprolalia* (the spontaneous utterance of socially objectionable words, such as obscenities and racial or ethnic slurs).

Features of Tourette's syndrome include:
- Multiple motor and one or more vocal tics present at some time during the disorder, although not necessarily simultaneously.
- The occurrence of tics many times a day (usually in bouts), nearly every day or intermittently throughout a span of more than one year.
- Periodic changes in the number, frequency, type, and location of the tics, and in the waxing and waning of their severity. Symptoms may disappear for weeks or months at a time.

Tardive dyskinesia

Tardive dyskinesia is a serious neurological disorder caused by the long-term use of traditional antipsychotic (neuroleptic) drugs. The new generation of atypical antipsychotic appears to cause tardive dyskinesia less frequently.

Tardive dyskinesia is characterized by repetitive, involuntary, purposeless movements. Features of the disorder may include grimacing, tongue protrusion, lip smacking, puckering and pursing of the lips, and rapid eye blinking. Rapid movements of the arms, legs, and trunk may also occur.

📕 Assessing children and adolescents
📕 Interventions in child and adolescent mental health

Further reading

Neuropsychiatry and Behavioral Neurology Explained. 2003. Elsevier Health Sciences: Philidelphia. Author: Mitchell AJ.

Sleep disorders

A sleep disorder, called somnipathy, is an interruption or disturbance in the usual sleep patterns of a person. Some sleep disorders can interfere with a person's mental and emotional function because they interfere with REM sleep (see below).

Normal sleep stages

Stage 1

This is experienced as falling asleep, and is a transition stage between wake and sleep. It lasts between one and five minutes and occupies approximately 2–5% of a normal night of sleep.

Stage 2

This follows stage one and is the 'baseline' of sleep. It is part of the 90 minute cycle (see below) and occupies approximately 45–60% of sleep.

Stage 3 and 4

Stage 2 sleep evolves into 'Delta' sleep after approximately 10–20 minutes and may last for 15–30 minutes. It is also called 'slow wave' sleep, because brain activity slows down dramatically. In most adults, these two stages are completed within the first two 90 minute sleep cycles or within the first three hours of sleep. Delta sleep is the 'deepest' stage of sleep and the most restorative.

Stage 5

Rapid eye movement (REM) sleep is a very active stage of sleep and composes 20–25% of a normal night's sleep. Breathing, heart rate, and brain wave activity quicken. Vivid dreams can occur.

Sleep cycles

A typical night's sleep has four or five cycles of these sequential stages, each lasting between 90–110 minutes. As the night progresses, the amount of time spent in Delta sleep decreases with a corresponding increase in REM sleep.

Insomnia

Insomnia is a difficulty in going to sleep and/or maintaining sleep. The term insomnia is often used to indicate all stages and types of sleep loss. Insomnia is a symptom, not a disorder.

Primary insomnia

Aetiology

Primary insomnia occurs in up to 10% of adults and up to 25% of elderly adults. It appears to be slightly more common in women. There may be a different cause of primary insomnia for each individual, but it often involves a preoccupation with the inability to sleep or excessive worry about sleep, which can cause the person to stay awake. Many people report that they sleep better away from home; suggesting that conditioning related to the bedroom has occurred. This can result in bouts of sleep while watching TV, being a passenger in a car, or other areas not associated with the bedroom.

Symptoms
The criteria for a diagnosis of primary insomnia includes a difficulty falling asleep, remaining asleep, or receiving restorative sleep for no less than one month. This disturbance in sleep must cause significant distress or impairment in social, occupational, or other important functions. It should not appear exclusively during the course of another mental or medical disorder, or when alcohol, medication, or other substances are being used.

Primary hypersomnia
Aetiology
Up to 5% of the population has hypersomnia at some point in their lives, and it is more prevalent in males. The causes can vary greatly, but often the symptoms begin before the age of 30, and continue to progress unless treated. Some research suggests that sleep disruptions during the night (such as breathing-related sleep disorders) result in a lack of REM sleep; so the person feels tired, despite the fact that they have slept through the night.

Symptoms
The criterion for a diagnosis of primary hypersomnia includes excessive sleepiness for at least one month; demonstrated by prolonged sleep during the night or excessive daytime sleep. The hypersomnia must cause significant distress or impairment for the individual, and it should not occur exclusively during another mental illness, medical condition, or substance use.

Narcolepsy
Narcolepsy is diagnosed when a person has repeated sudden occurrences of sleep for a period of at least three months. To be diagnosed with narcolepsy, at least one of the following must be present: cataplexy (brief episodes of sudden loss of muscle tone) and REM intrusions (REM sleep occurs at unexpected times and results in hallucinations or sleep paralysis). Symptoms caused by another mental disorder, a medical condition, or the use of substances must be ruled out.

Further reading

Charney, PR, Geyer, GD, Berry, RB. *Clinical Sleep Disorders.* Lippincott Williams & Wilkins. Philadelphia: 2004.
Hirshkowitz M, Patricia, B. *Sleep Disorders for Dummies.* For Dummies: 2004. New York.

Post-traumatic stress disorder (PTSD)

PTSD is a severe psychological disturbance following a traumatic event. The two key definitions as to what constitutes a traumatic event are:

ICD-10 definition	DSM-IV definition
A stressful event or situation . . . . of an exceptionally threatening or catastrophic nature which is likely to cause pervasive distress in almost anyone. Includes traumatic events such as rape, criminal assault, and natural catastrophe. Resulting in sudden changes in the social position or network of a person.	The traumatic event must have involved actual or threatened death or serious injury, or a threat to the physical integrity of self and others. The person's response to the traumatic event must have involved intense fear, helplessness, or horror.

Using these criteria, up to 80% of men and 75% of women may experience one traumatic event in their lifetime. Common events include the sudden death of a loved one, accidents, fire, flood, natural disasters, or being a witness to severe injury. PTSD is also referred to as Type 1 and Type 2 trauma.

Typical symptoms of PTSD are:
- Repeated reliving of the trauma in intrusive memories, 'flashbacks', or dreams.
- Persisting background sense of 'numbness'.
- Emotional blunting.
- Detachment from other people.
- Unresponsiveness to surroundings.
- Anhedonia (failure to enjoy positive emotional experiences).
- Avoidance of activities and situations reminiscent of the trauma.
- Fear and avoidance of cues that remind the sufferer of the original trauma.
- Autonomic hyperarousal with hypervigilance (constantly feeling that something awful is about to happen).
- Enhanced startle reaction.
- Insomnia.
- Anxiety and depression.
- Suicidal ideas.
- Excessive use of alcohol or drugs – may be a complicating factor.
- Rarely, there may be dramatic, acute bursts of fear, panic or aggression, triggered by stimuli arousing a sudden recollection and/or re-enactment of the trauma, or of the original reaction to it.

High risk groups for PTSD include:
- Those on active service in the armed forces.
- Refugees and asylum seekers.
- Victims of torture.
- People who have experienced traumatic events, including childhood experiences.

Helen Waldock, Health and Social Care Advisory Service

There is debate about the validity of a diagnosis of PTSD as a mental illness because:

- It excludes low magnitude stressors e.g. divorce, job loss, failing exams.
- Common events such as road traffic accidents and rape often lead to PTSD-type symptoms.
- Perpetrators of events, albeit unwillingly, can experience the same degree of symptoms as their victims.
- The emphasis on life threatening events, or on threats to physical integrity, makes it a fairly restrictive diagnosis.

Further Reading

Website: www.ptsdalliance.org

Semple D, Smyth R, Burns J, Darjee R, McIntosh A. *Oxford Handbook pf Psychiatry*. Oxford University Press: Oxford 2005.

Soli P, Williams MB. *The PTSD Workbook: simple effective techniques for overcoming traumatic stress symptoms*. New Harbinger Publication: 2002. Oakland.

Mental Health Act 1983

The Mental Health Act Code of Practice

At present, the Mental Health Act (England & Wales) 1983, covers the detention of patients into mental health services. The Code of Practice gives guidelines for best practice on the use of the Mental Health Act (MHA).[1]

The Code of Practice (COP)

Unlike the MHA, the COP does not have the force of the law behind it. But any service provider who deviates from the Code must have very good reasons for doing so, and these reasons may be subject to evidence in any legal proceedings.

The COP is useful for:
- Raising standards.
- Attracting resources.
- Clarifying responsibilities.
- Agreeing procedures, guidelines, and practices.
- Increasing and improving training.
- Setting objectives.
- Monitoring and evaluating practice.
- Preventing or resolving disputes between people.
- Raising awareness of patients' rights.
- Encouraging multidisciplinary work.
- Drawing up checklists.
- Pressing for reforms.
- Identifying discrepancies, deficiencies, malpractice and weaknesses.
- Familiarizing people with statutory duties.

📖 Working with the person who uses forensic services.

Patrick Callaghan, Professor of Mental Health Nursing, University of Nottingham & Nottinghamshire Healthcare NHS Trust

References

1 Department of Health. The Mental Health Act Code of Practice. HMSO: London, 2003.

Further reading

Dimond, BC, Barker, FH. *Mental Health Law for Nurses.* Blackwell Science: London, 1996.

Involuntary detention

At present, the detention of patients into mental health services is governed by the Mental Health Act (England & Wales) 1983. The table opposite outlines the main provisions of the Mental Health Act as they relate to involuntary detention.

Patrick Callaghan, Professor of Mental Health Nursing, University of Nottingham & Nottinghamshire Healthcare NHS Trust

Section number and purpose	Maximum duration	Can patient apply to MHRT?	Automatic MHRT hearing?	Can nearest relative apply to MHRT?	Do consent to treatment issues apply?
2 Admission and treatment	28 days, not renewable	Within first 14 days	No	No	Yes
3 Admission for treatment	6 mths. May be renewed for 6 mths, then annually	Within first 6 mths, then in each period 1 yr	Yes – at 6 mths, then every 3 yrs (yearly if under 16) if no application	No	Yes
4 Emergency admission for assessment	72 hrs. Not renewable but 2nd doctor can change to s2	Yes, but only if s4 is converted to s2	No	No	No
5(2) Doctors' holding power	72 hrs. Not renewable	No	No	No	No
5(4) Nurses' holding power	6 hrs. Not renewable, but doctor can change to 5(2)	No	No	No	No
7 Reception in guardianship	6 mths. May be renewed for 6mths, then yearly	Within first 6 mths, then in each period of 1 yr	No	No	No
16 Dr re-classifies the mental disorder	For the duration of the detention	Within 28 days of being informed	No	No	No

Section number and purpose	Maximum duration	Can patient apply to MHRT?	Automatic MHRT hearing?	Can nearest relative apply to MHRT?	Do consent to treatment issues apply?
18 Transfer from guardianship to hospital	6 mths. May be renewed for 6 mths, then annually	Within first 6 mths, then in each period	Yes – at 6 mths, then every 3yrs (yearly if under16) if no application	No	Yes
25 Restriction of discharge by nearest relative	Variable	No	No	Within 28 days of being informed	
25A Supervised aftercare	6 mths. May be renewed for 6 mths, then annually	6 mths May be renewed for 6 mths, then annually	No	Yes, if entitled to be informed, once in each period	No
135 Warrant to search for and remove patient	72 hrs. Not renewable	No	No	No	No
136 Police power in public places to remove person to place of safety	72 hrs. Not renewable	No	No	No	No

Further reading

Jones, R. *The Mental Health Act Manual*, 9th edn. Sweet & Maxwell: London, 2004.

Court orders

At present, the detention of patients into mental health services is governed by the Mental Health Act (England & Wales) 1983. The following are the main provisions of the Mental Health Act 1983 as they relate to involuntary detention for people referred from the justice system.

Patrick Callaghan Professor of Mental Health Nursing, University of Nottingham & Nottinghamshire Healthcare NHS Trust

Section number and purpose	Maximum duration	Can patient apply to MHRT?	Can nearest relative apply to MHRT?	Automatic MHRT hearing?	Do consent to treatment issues apply?
35 Remand to hospital for psychiatric report	28 days. May be renewed by court for further 28 days to maximum of 12 weeks	No	No	No	No
36 Remand to hospital for psychiatric treatment	28 days. May be renewed by court for further 28 days to maximum of 12 weeks	No	No	No	Yes
37 Guardianship order by court	6 mths. May be renewed for 6 mths, then annually	Within first 6 mths, then in each period	Within first year, then yearly	No	No
37 Hospital order by court	6 mths. May be renewed for 6 mths, then annually	In second 6 mths, then in each period	In second 6 mths, then in each period	If one has not been held the Hospital Managers refer to MHRT every 3 yrs	Yes
37/41 Restriction order by court	Variable	In second 6 mths, then annually	There is no nearest relative	If one has not been held the Home Secretary refers to MHRT every 3 yrs	Yes
38 Interim hospital order by court	12 weeks. May be renewed by 28 days at a time to maximum of 1 year	No	No	No	Yes

Section number and purpose	Maximum duration	Can patient apply to MHRT?	Can nearest relative apply to MHRT?	Automatic MHRT hearing?	Do consent to treatment issues apply?
45A Hospital and limited directions	Without limit of time	In first 6 mths, second 6 mths, then annually	No	If one has not been held the Home Secretary refers to MHRT every 3 yrs	Yes
46 Transfer to hospital of persons in custody during HM's pleasure	Without limit of time	Within first 6 mths, then in each period	No	If one has not been held the Home Secretary refers to MHRT every 3 yrs	Yes
47 Transfer to hospital of a person serving a prison sentence	6 mths. May be renewed for 6 mths, then annually	Within first 6 mths, then in each period	No	If one has not been held the Hospital Managers refer to MHRT every 3 yrs	Yes
47/49 Transfer from prison and restrictions	Restriction order expires on earliest date of release from prison	In second 6 mth period after transfer, then annually	There is no nearest relative	If one has not been held the Home Secretary refers to MHRT every 3 yrs	Yes
48 Transfer to hospital of other prisoners	Variable	Within first 6 mths, then in each period	No	If one has not been held the Home Secretary refers to MHRT every 3 yrs	Yes
136 Police power in public places to remove person to place of safety	72 hrs Not renewable	No	No	No	No

📖 Working with the person who uses forensic services

Further reading
Jones, R. *The Mental Health Act Manual*, 9th edn. Sweet & Maxwell: London, 2004.

Nurses' holding powers: Section 5(4)

At present, the detention of patients into mental health services is governed by the Mental Health Act (England & Wales) 1983. This chapter outlines the main provisions of Section 5(4): Nurses' holding powers.

📖 Code of professional practice and ethics

The use of Section 5(4)

Section 5(4) may be used by a registered mental nurse, or by a registered nurse who is trained in caring for people with learning disabilities, to detain an informal patient for a maximum period of 6 hours; where the detention is necessary for the health and safety of the patient or others, and where it is not possible for the Registered Medical Officer (RMO) to attend.

Issues for the nurse to consider in using section 5(4)

- If section 5(4) is used, the nurse must try to secure the attendance of the RMO as soon as possible, so that the patient can be assessed for detention under another section.
- Under section 5(5) of the Mental Health Act the nurse must make a report to management as soon as possible after using section 5(4).
- Patients must be informed of their rights under section 5(4) as soon as possible after it is used.
- If the RMO detains the patient under section 5(2), the 72-hour period of this detention starts from the time that the nurse made the report of detention under section 5(4).
- The nurse can make another report for a further six hours detention if the RMO has not arrived before the end of the six hours. However, this is against the spirit of the Act and should be discouraged. It may be possible for the RMO to nominate someone else to act on his or her behalf under section 5(3).
- Patients detained under section 5(4) cannot be given medication against their will, as this section is not covered by Part 4 of the Act governing consent to treatment issues. It might be possible to justify giving a patient medication under section 5(4), using common law powers.
- Section 5(4) can only be used when a person is an in-patient who is being treated for a mental disorder. It cannot be used on a person who is being treated in a general hospital for a physical illness, and who becomes mentally ill.

Patrick Callaghan, Professor of Mental Health Nursing, University of Nottingham & Nottinghamshire Healthcare NHS Trust

Further reading

Dimond, BC, Barker, FH. *Mental Health Law for Nurses*. Blackwell Science: London, 1996.
Jones, R. *The Mental Health Act Manual*, 9th edn. Sweet & Maxwell: London, 2004.

Mental Health Review Tribunals (MHRTs)

At present, the detention of patients into mental health services is governed by the Mental Health Act (England & Wales) 1983. People who are detained under the Mental Health Act are deprived of a fundamental liberty; systems are therefore in place for detained patients to appeal against their detention. They may appeal to the hospital managers under Section 23 of the Act, their nearest relative may appeal for their discharge, or they may appeal to a Mental Health Review Tribunal. 📖 Involuntary detention and 📖 Court Orders outline the rights of detained patients to appeal to a MHRT.

The composition of a MHRT is governed by specific rules. The panel has legal members, medical members, and members with knowledge of administration and social services. MHRT's are not public hearings, but could be public if the patient requests it. This section describes the role of the MHRT.

The Powers of a MHRT

The MHRT can discharge patients held under certain sections of the Mental Health Act. Patients under Section 2 must be discharged if the MHRT is satisfied that:

- They are not suffering from a mental disorder (as defined in Section 1 of the Act) that needs detention for assessment, or
- That the section is not justified in the interests of the health and safety of the patient or others.

The MHRT must discharge patients under sections other than Section 2, if it is satisfied that:

- The patient is not suffering from a mental disorder that needs detention for treatment, or
- Detention is not justified in the interests of the health and safety of the patient or others, or
- That the patient, if released would not be a danger to themselves or others.

MHRTs have discretionary powers to discharge patients even if the conditions outlined above are not satisfied. If they are not satisfied, then the MHRT must consider whether the treatment is likely to alleviate or prevent deterioration in the patient's condition; or if the patient is discharged, whether they are able to care for him or herself.

Patients can withdraw their appeal to the MHRT; and they can appeal to the High Court against the decision of the MHRT.

Patrick Callaghan, Professor of Mental Health Nursing, University of Nottingham & Nottinghamshire Healthcare NHS Trust

Procedures before a MHRT hearing

- An application to the MHRT must be made in writing.
- Patients should be informed of their rights, especially their right to legal representation.
- Patients should be given assistance to complete the application form and to seek legal representation.
- The patient's nearest relative should be informed of their right to attend the MHRT, and of their right to provide information to the tribunal in advance of the hearing.

📖 Working with advocacy services.

The role of the nurse

- To ensure the patient has appropriate knowledge about the application (and the tribunal).
- To assist the patient in finding legal representation.
- To provide a report for the MHRT if requested.
- To give evidence to the MHRT if required.

Further reading

Dimond, BC, Barker, FH. *Mental Health Law for Nurses.* Blackwell Science: London, 1996.
Jones, R. *The Mental Health Act Manual*, 9th edn. Sweet & Maxwell: London, 2004.

The Mental Health Act Commission (MHAC)

At present, the detention of patients into mental health services is governed by the Mental Health Act (England & Wales) 1983. The Mental Health Act Commission was established in 1983; it consists of Commissioners who are a mixture of lay-people, lawyers, doctors, nurses, social workers, psychologists, and other specialists.

The functions of the MHAC
- To keep under review the operation of the Mental Health Act 1983, in respect of patients liable to be detained under the Act.
- To visit and interview, in private, patients detained under the Act in hospitals and in mental nursing homes.
- To investigate complaints which fall within the Commission's remit.
- To review decisions to withhold the mail of patients detained in the High Security Hospitals.
- To appoint medical practitioners and others to give second opinions in cases where this is required by the Act.
- To publish and lay before Parliament a report every 2 years.
- To monitor the implementation of the MHA Code of Practice and propose amendments to ministers.

The Commission is also encouraged by the Secretary of State to advise on policy.

The role of Mental Health Act Commissioners
There are two types of commissioners who have different roles:

Local commissioners
- Visit detained patients.
- Examine their statutory records.
- Take up immediate issues on their behalf.
- Prioritize issues for action and decide how best to resolve them.
- Maintain supportive but objective relationships with providers at a local level.
- Take part in national visits on specific topics.

Area commissioners
- Coordinate the work of the MHAC within a Strategic Health Authority (SHA) or Welsh Region.
- Develop and maintain relationships with providers, social services departments, user groups, and all relevant agencies in relation to detained patients.
- Are responsible for collating, writing, and presenting annual reports to the boards of all providers.

Patrick Callaghan Professor of Mental Health Nursing, University of Nottingham & Nottinghamshire Healthcare NHS Trust

Commissioners are divided into four regional teams, each covering a different geographical area. Within each regional team, commissioners are allocated to a Strategic Health Authority or Welsh Region area. They aim to visit each hospital or unit in their area every 12 months and every ward within each hospital or unit every 18 months.

Members of the Commission have to meet detained patients. Meetings are undertaken by a single member of the Commission. They are usually held in private, with individual patients or clients.

The role of second opinion appointed doctors

When a detained patient is incapable of consenting or refusing to consent to treatment, the RMO responsible for the patient's care has a statutory responsibility to obtain a second opinion. This must be from an independent second doctor appointed by the Mental Health Act Commission, at times set by the Mental Health Act.

For non-consenting patients, a second opinion is required if medication is to be continued after the initial three months of treatment has expired. In the case of ECT, a second opinion is required at any time (Section 58 of the Act) for a non-consenting patient.

The Commission has a panel of approximately 150 consultants spread throughout England and Wales. They also appoint panels made up of doctors and other persons to validate treatments falling within the provisions of Section 57 (neurosurgery for mental disorder). In order to go ahead with this form of treatment, the patient must consent and the appointed panel – consisting of three persons (one doctor and two other persons) – must independently agree that the patient is able and willing to consent and that the treatment should be given.

Further reading

Jones, R. *The Mental Health Act Manual*, 9th edn. Sweet & Maxwell: London, 2004.
The Mental Health Act Commission website: www.mhac.org.uk

Aftercare under supervision (AUS)

At present, the detention of patients into mental health services falls under the auspices of the Mental Health Act (England & Wales) 1983.

Section 117(2) of the Mental Heath Act places a duty of care on PCTs, Trusts, or Social Services Departments to provide aftercare services for patients entitled to these services following discharge from hospital. This care is generally provided under CPA or the Care Programme Approach. But the provisions of section 117 apply only to patients who have ceased to be detained under Section 3. Under Section 25, aftercare under supervision (AUS) may be used to ensure that a patient receives the appropriate after-care required under Section 117.

📖 CPA
📖 Following through on programmes of care

Use of AUS

AUS is used for:
- Patients who have previously been detained for treatment.
- People who need suitable aftercare to prevent substantial risk of serious harm to themselves or others, or who are at risk of serious exploitation.

Prior to discharge, the patient must have a community responsible medical officer (RMO) assigned to them. This person is responsible for the patient's treatment after discharge. The patient must also have an identified supervisor who will act as their key worker under the CPA.

Guardianship can be used for a patient who needs aftercare, but who does not meet all of the criteria for AUS, Section 7.

AUS will end as soon as a patient is admitted to hospital under Section 3 or 37. AUS is suspended if a patient is admitted informally, or under Section 2.

Procedure for AUS

Aftercare arrangements must be drawn up as part of normal discharge planning.

Before the AUS order is made, the service provider responsible for the patient's care must make arrangements with the authorities who will be providing care once the patient is discharged.

The RMO who makes the supervision application is responsible for making sure that the existing and future care teams know about the arrangements for aftercare.

Duration of Aftercare Under Supervision

AUS begins when the patient leaves hospital and lasts for 6 months. It may be renewed for a further 6 months, then yearly.

Further reading

Jones, R. *The Mental Health Act Manual*, 9th edn. Sweet & Maxwell: London, 2004.

Department of Health and Welsh Office. Mental Health Act 1983 Code of Practice. DoH: London, 1999.

Patrick Callaghan Professor of Mental Health Nursing, University of Nottingham & Nottinghamshire Healthcare NHS Trust

The Mental Health (Care & Treatment) (Scotland) Act 2003

The Millan Principles

The new Act differs from the 1983 act principally in that it gives greater focus to the rights of the individual with mental disorders and their carers. It was developed in co-operation with all of those involved in mental health care, including patients and carers, professional or otherwise. The principles developed by the Millan Committee, although not addressed directly in all parts of the act have been the guiding principles for and have influenced much of the provision encompassed within the Act.

These principles are:
- Non-discrimination
- Equality
- Respect for Diversity
- Reciprocity
- Informal Care
- Participation
- Respect for Carers
- Least restrictive treatment options
- Benefit
- Child welfare

Within the Act the powers and responsibilities of Local Authorities have been increased in order to meet the requirements of patients and carers. The needs of informal carers are also specifically addressed within the act as are the needs for specific care provision for children with mental health problems.

Advance Statements

This is a provision within Part 18 of the act that allows the patient, when well, to prepare an Advance Statement setting out how they prefer to be treated, or not, if they become ill in the future. This statement is witnessed by an authorised person, under the terms of the Act and is in addition to previous requirements that those delivering care must have regard to the past and present wishes of the patient when doing so.

The Mental Health Tribunal and medical staff must send the Mental Welfare Commission (MWC) a written record of both the statement and how they plan to meet it. If for any reason they are unable to meet the requests in the statement they are required to give the MWC, in writing, the reasons for this failure. The patient is required to give a copy of this statement to any person who needs to know about it and keep list of these people. This would include carers, social worker, nurse and anyone else involved in their care.

The patient can also nominate a named person to look after their interests if they require treatment under the act, who has to be notified of and consulted on any change in status of treatment. The patient can also identify who should not be named person for them. If they do not nominate

Patricia A. McBride, University of Paisley

someone this will be done for them, automatically the primary carer or nearest relative. If these people do not wish to act in this capacity or are unavailable the Mental Health Officer (MHO) can apply to the Mental Health tribunal to have someone appointed.

The patient can, at any time, withdraw or change the Advance Statement and the named person.

Compulsory Treatment Order

The most significant change to detention and treatment arrangements under the new act is the Compulsory Treatment Order (CTO), which can be applied to both the hospital and any community setting. Its purpose is for the care and treatment of the patient to be delivered in the least restrictive environment appropriate to the patient needs.

Only the Mental Health Officer (MHO) can make the application and is obliged to do so on receiving two mental health reports indicating that it is necessary, even if the MHO does not agree. The reports must be from Approved Medical Practitioners, reach similar conclusions as to the mental state of the patient and have been carried out within 5 days of each other. The MHO then has a duty to:

• Identify the named person and explain to the patient their rights and status under the CTO;
• Notify the patient, the named person and the Mental Welfare Commission;
• Inform the patient about independent advocacy services and the right to appeal;
• Interview the patient and prepare a report.

The application for CTO is made to the Mental Health Tribunal and must contain a proposed care plan which must specify:

• The compulsory measures being sought;
• Medical treatment, community care services and any other form of treatment or service to be provided to the patient under the order;
• The name of the hospital whose manger will appoint the Responsible Medical Officer (RMO).

The CTO is initially applied for 6 months at which point it must be reviewed and can be applied for a further 6 months, thereafter to be reviewed at 12 monthly intervals. The patient's freedom should only be restricted as much as is necessary for their well-being and they have the right to appeal only after 3 months from the start date of the order.

In the case where further information is deemed necessary before applying a CTO and Interim CTO can be used. This would be in force for a 28 day period and if necessary for a further 28 days, up to a maximum of 56 days.

Medications

Drugs used in mental health treatment

Medicines used in mental health fall into four broad categories:
- Antipsychotics.
- Antidepressants.
- Mood stabilizers.
- Anxiolytics.

Antipsychotics

Typical or first-generation antipsychotics include chlorpromazine, haloperidol, sulpiride, trifluoperazine, and the depot injections flupentixol, fluphenazine, and pipotiazine and zuclopenthixol.

Atypical or second-generation antipsychotics include amisulpiride, aripiprazole, clozapine, olanzapine, quetiapine and risperidone (including the long-acting risperidone injection).

The main differences between the two groups are that the atypicals cause fewer extrapyramidal side-effects (EPSE) and fewer side-effects related to raised prolactin levels (hyperprolactinaemia), than the typical antipsychotics. EPSEs manifest as Parkinsonism (including tremor, stiff gait, mask-like face), dystonia (muscle stiffness), akathisia (restlessness) and the late onset movement disorder, tardive dyskinesia. Raised prolactin levels may cause reduced sexual libido, impotence in men, enlarged and painful breasts (gynaecomastia), lactation, and irregular or no menstruation.

However, as a group, the atypicals cause more weight gain and diabetes, the risk of metabolic syndrome (hypertension, diabetes, high cholesterol, central obesity).

Antidepressants

Selective serotonin reuptake inhibitors (SSRIs)
- SSRIs selectively block the reuptake of serotonin. They include fluoxetine, fluvoxamine, paroxetine, sertraline, citalopram.
- Common side-effects: nausea, anxiety, headache, sexual dysfunction (difficulty in reaching orgasm).

Tricyclic antidepressants (TCAs)
- Tricyclics block the reuptake of both serotonin and noradrenaline. They include amitriptyline, imipramine, dosulepin, lofepramine, nortriptyline, trimipramine.
- Common side-effects: anticholinergic side-effects (dry mouth, blurred vision, constipation), low blood pressure, dizziness, and sedation.

Monoamine oxidase inhibitors (MAOIs)
- MAOIs prevent the breakdown of noradrenaline and serotonin. Examples of MAOIs are phenelzine and tranylcypromine.
- Common side-effects are: low blood pressure, dizziness, blurred vision, insomnia, tremor, sexual dysfunction.

Shameen Mir, Chief Pharmacist, East London and the City Mental Health NHS Trust

- The danger with MAOIs is their potential to interact with other medicines, foods (containing tyramine) and alcoholic drinks.
- Other antidepressants include venlafaxine and duloxetine, also known as SNRIs (selective noradrenaline reuptake inhibitors), mirtazapine and reboxetine.

Mood stabilizers

Lithium

- Lithium treats mania as well as preventing future episodes of both mania and depression. It also reduces suicide.
- Common side-effects: fine tremor, weight gain, polydipsia, and polyuria.
- Common interactions: diuretics, non-steroidal anti-inflammatory drugs, haloperidol, carbamazepine, SSRIs, ACE inhibitors.

Carbamazepine

- Carbamazepine treats mania and prevents further episodes of mania and depression.
- Common side-effects: dizziness, drowsiness, ataxia, and nausea.
- Common interactions: increases the levels of most antidepressants, antipsychotics and anxiolytics.

Valproate

- This is available as sodium valproate (Epilim), valproic acid (Convulex) and semisodium valproate (Depokote). Valproate is effective in treating mania, although its efficacy in preventing future episodes is less certain.
- Common side effects: nausea, lethargy, confusion, and weight gain.

Anxiolytics

Benzodiazepines

- Benzodiazepines may be used for short-term treatment only. Examples include diazepam, lorazepam and clonazepam.
- Common side effects: sedation, amnesia, and dizziness.
- There is a danger of tolerance and addiction.

Antidepressants

Antidepressants may be used for the long-term treatment of anxiety. These include imipramine, paroxetine and venlafaxine (see above).

📖 Electro Convulsive therapy (ECT)
📖 Working with the client with a mood disorder
📖 Schizophrenia
📖 Depression
📖 Bipolar disorder
📖 Phobias

Safe administration of medicines

The right medicine(s) must reach the right patient, at the right dose, at the right time, via the right route. This is commonly known at the five Rs. Anything that prevents this will result in a medication error or clinical incident.

Principles for the administration of medicines

In exercising your professional accountability in the best interests of your patients, you must:

- Know the therapeutic use of the medicine to be administered, the normal dosage, its side-effects, precautions and contraindications.
- Be certain of the identity of the patient to whom the medicine is to be administered. This can be especially difficult in mental health as patients do not wear identification wrist bands.
- Be aware of the patient's care plan.
- Check that the prescription, and the label are clearly written and unambiguous, medicine is dispensed by a pharmacist.
- Check that prescribed medicines coincide with those listed on the relevant consent to treatment form (currently form 38 or 39).
- Consider the dosage, the method, route, and timing of administration, in the context of the condition of the patient and any co-existing therapies.
- Check the expiry date of the medicine to be administered.
- Check that the patient is not allergic to the medicine before administering it.
- Contact the prescriber, or another authorized prescriber without delay if contraindications to the prescribed medicine are discovered, if the patient develops a reaction to the medicine, or if assessment of the patient indicates that the medicine is no longer suitable.
- Make a clear, accurate and immediate record of all medicine administered, including those intentionally withheld or refused by the patient. Ensure that any written entries, and the signature, are clear and legible; it is also the coordinating nurses responsibility to ensure that a record is made when the task of administering medicine is delegated to a colleague.
- If you are supervising a student in the administration of medicines, clearly countersign the student's signature.

Management of medication incidents

- A medication incident occurs when something prevents the right patient receiving the right drug, at the right dose, at the right time via the right route.
- An incident must be reported immediately to the line manager or the employer.
- Omission of medication is an error unless it is accounted for.

Shameen Mir, Chief Pharmacist, East London and the City Mental Health NHS Trust

- Most organizations will have an incident reporting procedure – this must be followed.
- Make sure the patient is safe – carry out all necessary observations.
- The error must be documented in the medical and nursing notes.
- Inform the patient of the incident.

Further reading

Nursing and Midwifery Council. *Guidelines for the administration of medicines.* NMC: London January 2004.

Prescribing medication: general principles

- Medicines must be prescribed either by a medical practitioner or a secondary prescriber.
- Secondary prescribers (e.g. nurses, pharmacists, podiatrists, radiographers) may prescribe medicines for specific patients within an agreed clinical management plan.
- The prescribing of medicines should be based, whenever possible, on the patient's informed consent and their awareness of the purpose of the treatment.

The prescription

All prescriptions must:
- Be clearly written, typed, or computer-generated and be indelible.
- Clearly identify the patient for whom the medication is intended.
- Clearly specify the substance to be administered, using its generic or brand name where appropriate and its stated form, together with the strength, dosage, timing, frequency of administration, start and finish dates, and route of administration.
- Be signed and dated by the authorized prescriber.
- Not be for a substance to which the patient is known to be allergic, or is otherwise unable to tolerate.
- Where there is a requirement under the Mental Health Act for consent to be given concerning treatment, there should be a valid Form 38 or Form 39, reflecting the medication being administered.

Controlled Drugs

A prescription for controlled drugs must:
- Be in writing – and signed and dated by the person issuing it.
- Be in ink or otherwise indelible.
- Specify the address of the person issuing it, except in the case of an NHS or local health authority prescription.
- Specify (in the handwriting of the person issuing the prescription) the name and address of the person who it is for.
- Specify (in the prescriber's own handwriting) the dose to be taken.
- In the case of preparations, their form and, where appropriate, their strength must be specified. This can be either the total quantity of the preparation (in both words and figures), or the number (in both words and figures) of dosage units, as appropriate.
- In any other case, the total quantity (in both words and figures) of the controlled drug to be supplied must be recorded.
- If a prescription is for a total quantity intended to be dispensed by instalments, it must contain a direction specifying the amount of the instalments which may be dispensed and the intervals to be observed when dispensing.

Shameen Mir, Chief Pharmacist, East London and the City Mental Health NHS Trust

The National Institute for Health and Clinical Excellence has produced treatment guidelines[1] which include prescribing recommendations for the following mental illnesses:
- Schizophrenia.
- Depression.
- Eating disorder.
- Self harm.
- Anxiety.
- Violence.
- Post-traumatic stress disorder.
- Obsessive-compulsive disorder.

Maximum and minimum doses can be checked using the British National Formulary (BNF) that is available in all clinical areas and pharmacy departments.

Reference

1 Available at www.nice.org.uk

Further Reading

Pharmaceutical Society of Great Britain. Medicines, Ethics and Practice–A guide for pharmacists, 29th edn. Royal Pharmaceutical Press: July 2005.

Assessing and managing the side-effects of medication

Antidepressants

SSRIs

Nausea
- Assessment: direct questioning or observation e.g. patient may not feel like eating.
- Management: take medicine with food. If it persists, use an antiemetic.

Anxiety
- Assessment: direct questioning and visual observation.
- Management: if the patient is anxious to begin with, then start antidepressants at half the usual starting dose, and increase gradually. If the anxiety is severe, a short course of benzodiazepines can be prescribed.

Sexual dysfunction
- Assessment: direct questioning e.g. difficulty in reaching orgasm.
- Management: this is difficult to manage and usually requires changing treatment (e.g. mirtazapine, moclobemide, reboxetine).

Tricyclics

Dry mouth
- Assessment: direct questioning and observation e.g. fluid consumption.
- Management: it may wear off with time. Dose reduction where possible. Suck sugar free sweets, sip water (avoid sugary drinks). If it persists, use artificial saliva, or switch antidepressant to one with less anticholinergic side effects such as an SSRI. A persistent dry mouth can lead to an increase in dental caries.

Blurred vision
- Assessment: direct questioning.
- Management: may wear off with time. Dose reduction where possible. If it persists, switch antidepressant to one with less anticholinergic side effects such as an SSRI. Blurred vision cannot be corrected with optical glasses.

Constipation
- Assessment: direct questioning and observation of bowel motion.
- Management: dose reduction where possible. If severe, then treat with laxatives. Chronic constipation can lead to faecal impaction which can be life threatening. If it persists, switch antidepressant e.g. to an SSRI.

Dizziness
- Assessment: direct questioning, check postural drop.
- Management: may wear off with time. Reduce the dose where possible. If it persists, switch to an antidepressant with less anticholinergic side-effects such as an SSRI. Use cautiously with elderly patients because of the danger of falls.

Shameen Mir, Chief Pharmacist, East London and the City Mental Health NHS Trust

Antipsychotics
Extrapyramidal side-effects
Assessment can be done by observation, and more formally, using one of the rating scales below:

- **Simpson-Angus Scale (SAS):** for drug-induced acute extrapyramidal side-effects. It measures rigidity, tremor and pooling of saliva in the mouth.
- **Barnes Akathisia Scale (BAS):** for drug-induced akathisia.
- **Abnormal Involuntary Movement Scale (AIMS):** for tardive dyskinesia and other abnormal involuntary movements associated with antipsychotic drugs.

Management of extrapyramidal side-effects
- Dystonia: dose reduction, anticholinergic drugs. If it is severe or persistent, consider changing to an atypical antipsychotic.
- Parkinsonism: dose reduction, anticholinergic drug. If it is severe or persistent, consider changing to an atypical antipsychotic.
- Akathisia: dose reduction. Only use an anticholinergic drug if one of the above is present, otherwise, use propranolol. If it is severe or persistent, consider changing to an atypical antipsychotic.
- Tardive dyskinesia: this is difficult to manage. Consider switching to an atypical antipsychotic such as clozapine or olanzapine.

Prolactin–related side-effects
- Assessment: direct questioning. There may be reduced sexual libido, impotence in men, enlarged and painful breasts (gynaecomastia), lactation, and irregular or no menstruation.
- Management: these side-effects may respond to dose reduction. Switch to an atypical antipsychotic such as olanzapine, quetiapine, or aripiprazole.

Weight gain
- Assessment: by measuring baseline weight and subsequent monitoring.
- Management: diet and exercise programmes. Switching antipsychotics may be beneficial.

Diabetes
- Assessment: baseline fasting plasma glucose and subsequent monitoring.
- Management: switch antipsychotics e.g. to amisulpiride, aripiprazole, or clozapine. It is possible to continue treatment and treat the diabetes. Consider the risks and benefits in consultation with the individual.

Dry mouth, blurred vision, and constipation – see antidepressants.

Sedation

This can happen with twice daily dosing. If daytime sedation is a problem, consider giving all, or larger proportion of the dose at night.

📖 Electroconvulsive therapy (ECT)
📖 Working with the client with a mood disorder
📖 Schizophrenia
📖 Depression

Further reading

Taylor, D, Paton, C, Kerwin, R. *Prescribing Guidelines*, 8th edn. Taylor & Francis, The South London and Maudsley NHS Trust, and Oxleas NHS Trust: 2005.

Nurse prescribing

Nurse prescribing has been evolving for many years. It is intended to make services more responsive to the needs of service users and to make better use of nurses' existing skills. Research into forms of nurse prescribing in the United States suggests that nurse prescribing can be as safe as medical prescribing, and may be preferred by service users.

Educational preparation

The Nursing and Midwifery Council has defined competencies to be met over a course that contains at least 26 days of theory and 12 days of supervised learning in practice with a doctor. Mental health nurses must be supervised by consultant psychiatrists throughout their clinical placement regardless of the setting, as general practitioners do not have the expertise necessary in prescribing psychiatric medication. Many employing organizations arrange additional training to ensure competence in prescribing psychotropic medication, e.g. psychopharmacology modules.

Types of nurse prescribing

Nurses with a prescribing qualification can either act as a supplementary prescriber for any medication, or as an independent prescriber for any licensed medication, apart from controlled drugs. Nurses should only prescribe in areas for which they are competent.

Supplementary prescribing is a voluntary relationship between an independent prescriber (usually a doctor although this could be a nurse practitioner) and the supplementary prescriber (nurse), to implement an agreed clinical management plan (CMP) with the service user's agreement. The nurse can prescribe within the parameters of the CMP which must state the conditions under which the medication can be changed or altered.

Key factors necessary for supplementary prescribing:
• Communication between prescribing partners.
• Access to shared patient records (e.g. CPA).
• Service user to be an equal partner in their care.

Independent prescribing is where the nurse practitioner takes responsibility for the clinical assessment of the service user, establishing a diagnosis and the clinical management required, as well as taking responsibility for prescribing where necessary.

Utilising nurse prescribing

In order to prescribe safely and effectively, nurse prescribers need:
• Ongoing supervision.
• Use of their qualification to the benefit of service users.
• Opportunities to prescribe, and policies to support prescribing, including access to a budget.
• Maintain competence in line with the national frameworks.
• Work within the local reporting and recording policies and protocols.

Dr Neil Brimblecombe, Director of Mental Health Nursing, Department of Health & National Institute of Mental Health in England

Nurse supplementary prescribing is being used mainly in community settings and in specialist clinics, e.g. for early dementia. A few projects have been established in inpatient settings. Independent prescribing in mental health settings is untried at the time of publication, but is likely to be developed in all specialist areas of practice from spring 2006.

Further reading

Brimblecombe, N, Parr, A, Gray, R. Medication and mental health nurses: developing new ways of working. *Mental Health Practice* **8**(5): 12–14, 2005.
National Prescribing Centre. Improving mental health services by extending the role of nurses in pre-scribing and supplying medication: Good practice guide. NPC: Liverpool, 2005.

Chapter 9

Culture

Culturally capable mental health nursing

Mental health nurses play an important part in delivering equality in mental health services, through culturally capable practice. But there is widespread evidence that people from black and minority ethnic (BME) groups do not feel that the care they receive is equal, equitable, and sensitive to their needs.

What is culture?

Culture is a shared set of learned behaviours, values, beliefs, norms, assumptions, perceptions, customs, social interactions, and the world-view of a particular group.[1]

What is cultural capability?[1]

- *Awareness and respect* – for the ideas, beliefs, values, customs, expressions, and world-view of people from different races, ethnicities and cultures.
- *Willingness* – to work towards achieving capability.
- *Ability* – to see each person as an individual with needs, desires, and aspirations, that may be moulded by their culture, race, or ethnicity.

Framework of values for mental health and race equality

The National Institute of Mental Health in England identified the following framework of values for mental health practice:

- Recognition of the role of values in all areas of practice.
- Raising awareness of the values involved in different situations and how they impact upon practice.
- Respect for the diversity of users' values.
- Respect for diversity within mental health care that is user-centred, recovery oriented and multidisciplinary.

Values underlying cultural capability[1]

- *Awareness* – of your own value base, level of comfort with diversity, and personal biases.
- *Acceptance* – of difference (knowing that it does not mean inferiority), accepting your own and others' limitations, learning from others and making amends when necessary.
- *Knowledge* – the need to be learning at all times and the need to increase your knowledge of diversity.
- *Flexibility* – in handling unexpected situations.

Patrick Callaghan, Professor of Mental Health Nursing, University of Nottingham & Nottinghamshire Healthcare NHS Trust

A culturally capable mental health nurse will:

- Increase his/her own multicultural understanding – be aware of his/her own biases.
- Assess the extent to which people are oriented to their culture e.g. not all people belonging to the same ethnic group will be oriented to the same culture.
- Explore/assess how culture relates to thoughts, feelings, and behaviour.
- Demonstrate cultural sensitivity through understanding different experiences.
- Respect cultural norms in communication styles.
- Be aware of and avoid stereotyping.
- Ask, listen and respect.
- Be flexible – accommodate individual needs as far as possible.
- Respect and accept diversity.

📖 Transcultural nursing

References

1 Allot, P. Celebrating Cultural Diversity: Developing Cultural Capability. NIMHE: University of Wolverhampton, 2005.

Further reading

Department of Health. Delivering Race Equality in Mental Health Care: An action plan for reform inside and outside services, DoH: London, 2005. Available at www.dh.gov.uk

Working with people from different cultural and ethnic groups

Mental health nurses often work in multicultural settings and interact with people from different cultural and ethnic groups. People within these groups often behave and communicate in different ways.

Communication issues

When working with people from different cultural and ethnic groups communication issues may arise due to:

- *Rules* – groups have different rules for communication.
- *Language* – different groups often have their own language and dialect.
- *Motivation* – factors that drive communication such as rules, rituals may vary.
- *Ideals and values* – different beliefs underpin communication.
- *Cooperation and competition* – communication may be driven by these goals.
- *Collectivism and individualism* – communication may be directed at promoting the collective or the individual good.
- *Greetings and other rituals* – different groups have different rituals and ways of greeting each other e.g. handshakes, kissing.

Communication styles

Different cultural and ethnic groups have different styles of communication. The following issues may arise:

- Cultural context of language – the influence of culture on language varies.
- Self-disclosure – the meaning, use, and nature of self-disclosure varies among different groups.
- The preservation of face (i.e. not humiliating someone in front of others) is important in certain groups e.g. Chinese and Japanese people.
- The use and meaning of silence varies with different cultures.
- Varieties of truthfulness (i.e. respect for truth varies in different cultures).
- Complimenting and responding – may take different forms.
- Non-verbal behaviour has different meanings in different cultures.

The role of the mental heath nurse

- Increase one's own multicultural understanding – be aware of one's own biases.
- Assess the extent to which people are oriented to their culture e.g. not all people belonging to the same ethnic group will be oriented to the same culture.
- Explore/assess how culture relates to thoughts, feelings, and behaviour.
- Demonstrate cultural sensitivity through understanding different experiences.

Patrick Callaghan, Professor of Mental Health Nursing, University of Nottingham & Nottinghamshire Healthcare NHS Trust

- Respect cultural norms in communication styles.
- Beware of and avoid stereotyping.
- Ask, listen, and respect. Avoid using husbands or children as interpreters; in many cultures it is unacceptable to talk about intimate matters in front of family members.
- Be flexible – try to accommodate individual needs as far as possible.

📖 Transcultural nursing

Further reading

Department of Health. Delivering Race Equality in Mental Health Care: An action plan for reform inside and outside services, DoH: London, 2005. Available at www.dh.gov.uk

Fernando, S. *Cultural diversity, mental health and psychiatry: the struggle against racism.* Brunner-Routledge: Hove, 2003.

Sexuality and mental health – a research study

The area of sexuality and people with mental health problems is under-researched with one study giving direct guidance to mental health nurses.

Study aims

In 2005 a study by McCann[2] aimed to identify sexual and relationship needs as perceived by users of mental health services who were living in the community. The objective of this mixed methods study was to discover service users' past and present sexual experiences and to elicit hopes and aspirations for the future. Potential obstacles to sexual expression were highlighted through an exploration of subjective experiences of the issues that were important to service users.

Sample and context

A total of thirty people with a medical diagnosis of schizophrenia agreed to be interviewed at a clinic in North London, where they regularly attended to receive depot medication.

Data collection

Data were collected through:
- A questionnaire relating to demographic characteristics.
- An interview schedule incorporating the determinant factors of sexual behaviour through life.[3]
- Relevant sections of the Camberwell Assessment of Need.
- A semi-structured interview designed specifically for the study.

Analysis

Computer software packages were used to analyse both the quantitative and the qualitative data.

Findings

The findings reveal that people had clear ideas about what constituted a fulfilling intimate relationship. A majority of participants identified sex and relationship needs, and aspired to having relationships in the future. Obstacles were highlighted and these included: medication issues, body image, stigma and discrimination, support and the opportunity to discuss concerns, and access to family planning services or sexual and relationship therapy. People seemed comfortable about sharing details of intimate experiences during the interviews – none had to be prematurely terminated. A model of psychosexual care was proposed that includes rigorous methods of engagement, assessment, intervention, and evaluation strategies.

Scott Durairaj, Mersey Care NHS Trust

Role of the mental health nurse

Discussion of thoughts, feelings, and beliefs in relation to sexual aspects of health care is a challenging feature of nursing practice that needs sensitivity, confidence, a shared language, comprehension, and care Other challenges are presented in terms of education and professional role development such as: addressing inadequate knowledge of sexuality, exploring and modifying negative attitudes to sexuality, reducing discomfort with sexuality, and examining perceptions about the legitimacy of sexuality within nursing roles.

📖 Sexual disorders – female
📖 Sexual disorders – male
📖 Sexual disorders – female and male

References

2 McCann, E. Exploring sexual and relationship possibilities for people with psychosis – a review of the literature. *Journal of Psychiatric and Mental Health Nursing* **10**(6), 640–9, 2003.
3 Pfeiffer, R, Davis, G. Determinants of sexual behaviour in middle and old age. *Journal of the American Geriatric Society* **20**: 151–8, 1972.

Sexuality (sexual orientation) and mental health

Sexual orientation refers to the sex, sexes, gender, or genders to which a person is attracted and which form the focus of a person's loving or erotic desires, fantasies, and natural feelings. Other terms 'sexual preference' and 'sexual inclination' have related meanings. Some believe sexuality is fixed early in life while others believe sexuality is fluid and reflecting preference and choice. The term sexual orientation may also refer to the 'individuality' of a person, either by choice or as an expression of an inner attribute.

The majority of mental health professionals, backed by nearly 40 years of research, believe that it is possible to develop a happy and productive life in the context of a lesbian, bisexual, or gay ('les-bi-gay') sexual orientation, identity, and lifestyle. DSM IV no longer lists homosexuality as a mental illness. The only diagnostic reference to homosexuality in the manual relates to 'persistent and marked distress about sexual orientation' and it is the distress that characterizes the disorder, not the orientation itself. The desire to have sex is one of the basic drives of human behaviour.

The NHS Plan and many other NHS drivers for change are committed to a standard of equal access to, and equity of treatment in health care services. Currently, many lesbian, gay, and bisexual service users' experiences fall far short of this standard. Mental health workers sometimes fail to acknowledge same sex partners and their families. Ignoring a service user's partner can result in them not participating in the care of the ill person. It is best practice to involve those closest to the service users, who have knowledge of the service user's own wishes.

Next of kin

There is widespread misunderstanding about the term 'next of kin'. In a health care setting, this term has a very limited legal meaning; it relates to the disposal of a person's belongings to blood relations, if they have died intestate. But the term is also used in a number of other different ways – many service users think it means someone whose relationship to them has legal recognition. So asking for a person's 'next of kin' may confuse them, and is unlikely to give you the information you need.

For those patients who are detained under the Mental Health Act 1983 (and this is a minority of service users receiving help from mental health care providers), the issue of next of kin is often confused with the role of the 'nearest relative'. The role of the 'nearest relative' is to advocate on behalf of a service user. In the past, it has been difficult for same sex partners to gain recognition as the nearest relative. But in a recent case brought under the Human Right Act, a lesbian was successful in gaining recognition for her partner as her nearest relative (a partnership is defined as living with another person as husband or wife for 6 months or longer).

Dr Eddie McCann, City University, London

The Civil Partnership Act became law in December 2005. This act gives same sex couples the opportunity to legally register their relationship. Once registered, these couples will have similar rights to a heterosexual married couple (in terms of financial and legal matters). For more information see 'Get Hitched, a guide to civil partnerships' available free from www.stonewall.org.uk.

Where a service user is not treated under the Mental Health Act, the same considerations apply as elsewhere in the NHS. There is no limit to who may be selected as nearest relative or 'next of kin'. The decision should be the service user's choice; it could be their partner or a friend.

The Adults with Incapacity (Scotland) Act 2000, expressly recognizes a same sex partner as the nearest relative.

📖 Sexual disorders – female
📖 Sexual disorders – male
📖 Sexual disorders – female and male

Older people

Mental health disorders common in later life

Older people can be subject to the whole range of mental health disorders, (📖 Chapter 6, Common mental disorders). The two most common are dementia and depression.

Both these conditions have the potential for significantly reducing quality of life, dignity, and independence for the older person. Effective assessment and intervention by mental health nurses can make a difference in supporting the older person to be independent, and to have a life that is worth living.

Dementia

The term dementia is descriptive, and covers a global deterioration in mental function due to brain disease. It is progressive and chronic. Deterioration may be seen in:

- Memory.
- Thinking.
- Orientation.
- Comprehension.
- Calculation.
- Learning capacity.
- Language.
- Judgement.
- Emotional control.
- Social behaviour.
- Motivation.

These losses can have a powerful negative effect upon the person and their family. There is no cure for dementia, but effective and timely intervention from nurses and other professionals can help maintain an individual's psychological and physical functioning, and their social networks and relationships.

Prevalence of dementia

In a population of people in their late 60s, 1% might be diagnosed as having dementia. There is a steep increase with advancing age; 33% of 90 year olds might be expected to have dementia.

Depression

Depression in older people has all the characteristics as described in 📖 Depression. However some symptoms are distinct in older people.
📖 Working with the person with a mood disorder

Symptoms of depression more common in old age

- Complaints related to bodily, rather than emotional functioning.
- Loss and reduced ability to take pleasure in activities.
- Ideas of guilt, worthlessness, death, and suicide.
- Agitation.

Soo Moore, City University, London

- Decline in self-care.
- Deliberate self-harm.
- Suicide.

Symptoms of depression less common in old age

- Tiredness.
- Sleep disturbance.
- Weight loss.

Depression is treatable. Antidepressant medication, combined with talking therapies such as counselling, group therapy, life review, and social support, usually return the person to normal mood.

Prevalence of depression

In a population of people aged over 65 years, one would expect between 10–15% to exhibit some depressive symptoms; 3% may be diagnosed as having a severe depression.

Further reading

Jacob, R, Oppenheimer, C (eds.). *Psychiatry in the Elderly*, 3rd edn. Oxford University Press: Oxford, 2002.

Age-sensitive mental health nursing

Nursing older people with mental health problems requires a complex portfolio of skills, knowledge, motivation, values, and beliefs. Above all, the role requires the nurse to feel and display warmth, genuineness, and respect towards an undervalued group within society.

Working with older people is challenging and complex, as in old age people are more likely to have a multitude of pathologies. For example, a person of 85 years, besides having dementia, may well have diabetes, hypertension, and arthritis. The effective mental health nurse has to respond to all these needs when planning care.

Person-centredness

Person-centredness is a concept that is central to Government policy and clinical practice. Kitwood[1] has outlined the key features of offering person-centred care:

- Entering the patient's frame of reference – understanding where the person is in time and place and using this as vehicle to establish a dialogue.
- Non-judgemental acceptance of the uniqueness of the individual – ensuring actions and non verbal communication are not patronizing.
- Seeing the person as a whole.
- Having a positive view of human nature.
- Recognizing the importance of feelings and emotions.
- Recognizing the importance of interpersonal relationships.
- Valuing authenticity in relationships – being honest and sincere in interactions with older people.
- A non-directive approach- allowing the older person to make their own decisions.

These features are seen as a basis for structuring the assessment, planning, and delivery of nursing care for older people. They are the underpinning principles for the delivery of health and social care. Person-centredness is outlined in standard two of the National Service Framework for Older People.[2]

Context of nursing

The mental health nurse may offer a service to older people and their families in a variety of settings. In an inpatient setting the nurse lives alongside patients, and shares the ordinariness of life, supporting them in performing intimate personal activities. Trust may be built up through effective therapeutic relationships.

Families may derive support from a community mental health nurse who can broker for services, offer emotional support, and teach coping skills. Nurses working in any setting can use a range of therapeutic interventions to enable the older person to be fully engaged in life.

Soo Moore, City University, London

References

1 Kitwood, T. *Dementia Reconsidered: The person comes first.* Open University Press: Buckingham, 1997.
2 Department of Health. *National Service Framework for Older People.* The Stationary Office: London, 2001.

Communicating with the older adult

Effective communication is an essential feature of the mental health care of older people. Nurses have to be aware of their verbal and non-verbal communication. Often, depression, dementia, and sensory impairments form barriers to effective verbal communication, and the message is more easily conveyed by non-verbal means.

Effective communication with older people can be achieved by:
- Keeping your posture relaxed.
- Moving slowly and deliberately when within four feet of the older person.
- Not moving your hands or arms into an older person's intimacy circle.
- Ensuring you make your presence known before you touch a person – approaching from the rear and suddenly touching them can cause alarm.
- Having your eyes at the same level as theirs when talking with older people – crouch or kneel if talking to a person sitting in a wheelchair.
- Keeping your voice level, even, and calm.
- Establishing how the person wishes to be addressed and then using this name or title in interactions.
- Maintaining eye contact whilst you are talking.
- Using short sentences, repeating key words if necessary.
- Asking only one question at a time.
- Allowing the person time to respond.
- Giving only one instruction at a time – break down a complex request into simple steps.
- Checking that the person has understood.
- Ensuring that you are demonstrating listening by head nodding and responses.
- Ensuring that if a hearing aid is used it is turned on, in the appropriate ear, and has a working battery.
- Ensure that, if spectacles are worn, the person is wearing their own spectacles, the prescription is current, they are clean and appropriate. For example, not wearing reading glasses whilst eating lunch.

📖 Communication

Soo Moore, City University, London

Further reading

Killick, J, Allan, K. *Communication and the care of people with dementia*, Open University Press: Maidenhead, 2002.

Reality orientation

Reality orientation is a therapeutic approach to working with people with dementia. The aim is to provide individuals with the opportunity to use their retained abilities to strengthen weakened skills and to relearn others.

Group approach

Reality orientation is organized using a group of five or six members, with two therapists or group leaders. Simple material is used to stimulate participants to think about their relationships in order to maintain them. The main topics for discussion are introductions, time, date, weather, and location. The aim is to help the person to be oriented in time, place, and person. Once the group has been established it can move on to activities that promote interpersonal relationships, using humour or reminiscence for example.

24 hour reality orientation

In this approach, rather than rehearsing orienting information in a group setting, the carer uses opportunities in real life during everyday activities or when delivering personal care to repeat or provide information. Activities might include quizzes, games, or newspaper discussions. This is combined with extra aids in the environment such as large clocks, message boards, colour coded signing, and furniture arrangements.

Monitoring

Baseline observations are recorded before commencing reality orienteering and then repeated at regular intervals, so that quite small improvements can be recognized over time.

Soo Moore, City University, London

Further reading

Holden, UP, Woods, RT. Reality orientation: psychological approaches to the confused elderly. Churchill Livingstone: Edinburgh, 1995.

Reminiscence therapy

Reminiscence therapy uses the normal human activity of revisiting past times and events. In a therapeutic setting this is organized in a systematic way, and aims to provide a device to stimulate individuals to engage in social interaction. Revisiting former experiences may help to validate people by stimulating positive emotions associated with their past experience.

Coleman (1986) suggests that there may be three aspects of reminiscence:
- *Simple reminiscence* – when the person recalls the past and from this, derives a source of strength and esteem in the present.
- *Informative reminiscence* – when recollections are used to pass on knowledge.
- *Life review* – this involves analysis of aspects of one's life in order to achieve integration in the face of death.

Reminiscence therapy is usually conducted in institutional settings such as residential homes and day centres, as a facilitated group activity. Groups can be centred around:
- Music and sound recordings.
- Photographs and films.
- Outings.
- Practical activities such as cooking or gardening.
- Storytelling.
- Taste, touch, and smell.
- Drawing, painting, and collage.
- Handling objects – often artefacts that are symbolic of past times.
- Drama.

Soo Moore, City University, London

Further reading

Bornat, J (ed.). Reminiscence reviewed: perspectives, evaluations, achievements. Open University Press: Buckingham, 1993.

Coleman, PG. Ageing and reminiscence processes: social and clinical implications. Wiley: Chichester, 1986.

Validation therapy

Validation therapy has been defined by Feil as 'a therapy for communicating with very old people who are diagnosed as having Alzheimer's disease and related dementias'.[3] Validation suggests a way of classifying the behaviours of disoriented older people. It further suggests forms of communication to match the stages of dementia.

Validation offers the confused older person an empathetic listener, a non judgemental approach, and an acceptance of their reality.

Essential techniques of validation
- Centering – the care-giver uses techniques to give their full attention to the patient.
- Using non-threatening factual words to build trust.
- Rephrasing – repeating the essence of what the person has said back to them.
- Polarity – asking the patient to think about worst case scenarios to relieve their anxiety.
- Imagining the opposite – can lead to the recollection of a familiar solution.
- Reminiscing.
- Maintaining genuine, close eye contact.
- Using ambiguity – exploring ambiguous statements by using open questions and using pronouns.
- Using a clear, low, loving tone of voice.
- Observing and matching the person's motions and emotions (mirroring).
- Linking the patient's behaviour with the unmet human need.
- Identifying and using the patient's preferred sense for communication e.g. sight or hearing.

Soo Moore, City University, London

Reference

3 Feil, N. The Validation Breakthrough: simple techniques for communicating with people with Alzheimer's type Dementia. Health Professionals Press: Baltimore, 1993.

Leadership

Developing effective teams

Every team, regardless of the wider organizational context in which it sits, will have a unique team dynamic, an identity, and a micro-culture. Although each team will present differently, all teams require some common principles to be applied in order for them to be developed to their maximum potential.

Important areas to consider

There are three important areas to consider when developing a team. These are:
- The wider organization.
- The purpose and business of the team.
- The aptitudes, behaviours, experience, and skills contained within the team.

The wider organization

In order to develop a team, the boundaries and characteristics of the wider organization need to be clearly understood. This provides the framework within which a team needs to work. These are as follows:
- **The culture** – this incorporates the expressed aims and objectives, philosophy and mission of the organization as a whole. It defines the purpose and value base of the entire enterprise (📖 Culturally capable mental health nursing, 📖 Working with people from different cultural and ethnic groups).
- **The structure** – this includes the systems, hierarchy, and processes or rules that the organization has put into place in order to achieve its overarching purpose.
- **The lived experience** – this is the unspoken and unwritten belief systems that actually exist. It also includes the behaviors that are enacted within the organization. Sometimes, the lived experience may differ from the more formal philosophies expressed by the wider organization.

The purpose and business of a team

A successful team will have clarity surrounding the following:
- Its goals and purpose.
- Its agreed common approach to achieving its goals and purpose.
- Its mutual sense of joint accountability.
- Its united interdependence where each role and function is reliant on the effective functioning of the team as a whole.

Androulla Johnstone, Chief Executive, Health and Social Care Advisory Service

The aptitudes, behaviors, experience, and skills contained within the team

A team should be more that the sum of its collective parts. A team that is motivated and working well understands how to utilize the skills base of each of its individual members. In order to develop the team as a whole, together with the skills of its individual members, the aptitudes, behaviours, experience, and skills contained within the team need to be fully understood. If teams are to be developed to meet their full potential, the following aspects must be understood:

• Aptitudes for carrying out certain functions may be held by certain individuals. How should a team respond to this? Should the team allow one person to become a specialized resource or should the whole team continue to hone their skills in this area?

• Working in a team environment can be a challenge. Everyday stresses and tensions can lead to hindering and unhelpful behaviours. For a team to develop in a useful manner hindering and unhelpful behaviours need to be identified and mitigated against.

• All teams will contain a mixture of experience and skills. Most professional teams are assembled with their individuals already fit for purpose. The art of developing a team is to grow skills and experience so that innovation and flexibility are encouraged.

Teams do not work in isolation. To develop an effective team it is important to understand the macro culture of the wider organization, the goals and purpose of the team, and the ability of the individuals in the team to be efficient and effective.

Leading effective teams

A team is 'a small group of people with complementary skills committed to a common purpose and a set of specific performance goals'. The way a team is led will have a direct impact upon its potential success. An effective leader will require a set of specific skills.

The skills of an effective leader could include:

A commitment to people

- Ensuring the developmental needs of team members are met.
- Utilizing tools such as appraisal, mentoring, coaching, and consistent supervision.
- Ensuring the individual development of team members – this benefits them and the team.

Enthusiasm

- Developing a vision that is known by all, and encouraging team members to buy into it.
- Keeping morale high by acknowledging the expertise within the team and ensuring it is used for everyone's benefit.

Ability to take responsibility

- Team leaders are tested under pressure.
- A leader's role is to take challenges, to ensure that their team services them and that roles are delegated appropriately.

Ability to give praise and constructive feedback

Giving constructive feedback honestly but without inflicting damage or hurt is a skill, particularly when the message may be difficult for the other person to hear.

One technique used is the 'criticism sandwich'. The team leader first highlights what went well, then brings in areas for development, and ends on a positive achievement.

A commitment to developing your team

All teams will experience change as new members join, additional skills are added, and the goals of the team change.

The ingredients of an effective team are created by the combination of a skilled team leader, willing team members who are supported and developed, and a set of defined and agreed shared goals. This combination is likely to leave team members feeling good about the team they are in.

Team building has been described as 'like coaching, but for a group'.[1] Whether team building is soft (shared meals, sporting events) or hard (inter-team learning, team away days), it is a useful tool to build morale and relationships.

Finally, it is amazing what you can accomplish if you do not care who gets the credit (President Harry S Truman, (1884–1972).

Cathe Gaskell, Deputy Chief Executive, Nightingale House, London

Reference

1 Belbin R, Meredith. *Management Teams – why they succeed or fail.* 2003, Elsevier Science & Technology Oxford.

Further reading

Covey, R, Stephen. *First Things First.* Simon & Schuster: 1994. London.

Neil, J. What are Team Building Definitions, 2004. Available at: www.wilderdom.com/teambuilding

Katzenbach, J. *The Wisdom of Teams: Creating a High Performance Organisation.* McGraw Hill Publishing Co. 2005. London.

Leading an empowered organization

What is leadership?

Leadership is about direction, giving people a sense of purpose that inspires and motivates them to achieve. Leadership is also about a relationship between people – leaders and followers – that is built on shared values and trust.

Successfully leading an organization requires a complex balance between developing the people in it, managing its resources effectively, and ensuring people sign up to and progress toward a shared vision. Most successful leaders have a well defined sense of their own strengths and weaknesses. They do not try to be all things to all people. They are genuine and they develop a wide range of interpersonal skills.

What skills make a leader?

According to Mary Bast, leadership skills are based on leadership behaviours.[2] She believes skills alone do not make a leader, but style and behaviours do.

Top five leadership behaviours

- Integrity.
- Fairness.
- Prioritizing your work.
- Being positive with yourself and others.
- Listening to people.

All empowered organizations try to build leadership capacity, as good leadership can promote substantial organizational performance. Poor leadership has the opposite effect, resulting in high turnover and absenteeism.

There are as many styles of leadership as there are leaders. The following combination of styles will be adapted to suit the organizational needs and existing style of the leader.[3]

What successful leaders accomplish

Successful leaders lead positively charged or empowered organizations; they deliberately seek to increase the flow of positive emotions within an organization. Studies, show that leaders who share positive emotions have staff who exhibit:[4]

- A more positive mood.
- Enhanced job satisfaction.
- Greater engagement and improved performance.

Cathe Gaskell, Deputy Chief Executive, Nightingale House, London

Finally, a great leader recognizes the input of others to the organization's overall services – large and small. All input and effort should be acknowledged regularly. *'I praise loudly. I blame softly'* (Catherine the Great – 1729–1796) is an excellent motto for aspiring leaders, even today.

Leadership styles in an empowered organisation	
Visionary	Focusing on long term objectives and possibilities whilst developing a picture of the future. They encourage the teams around them to contribute to the vision. And they hold the values of the organization within the vision.
Mentor	Healthy mentors are unconditionally caring leaders who derive satisfaction from encouraging the development of others. They support training throughout the organization.
Democrat	Ensuring many voices are heard, placing a high value on inclusive communication. They use a range of mediums to get their message across, are highly visible and 'walk the talk'.
Diplomat	Bringing cooperation to the work environment, they enjoy building consensus and developing a shared sense of direction. Looking for agreement and cohesion where possible.
Innovators	Are vital to the health of an organization. They encourage risk taking, support new ideas, and they are not bound by tradition. They enjoy challenging the status quo.

References

2 Bast, M. Breakthroughs with the Enneagram, 1995. Available at:
www.internationalenneagram.org

3 Clinton D, Rath, T. *How full is your bucket?* Gallup Press Princeton New Jerey: 2005. See also:
www.bucketbook.com

4 Chapman, A. 1995–2005. See: www.businessballs.com

Further reading

Conchie, B. The seven demands of leadership: What separates great leaders from the rest?, 2005.
    Available at: www.gmj.gallup.com

Covey, R. Stephen *Principle-Centred Leaderships*. Simon & Shuster: 2004. London

Managing effective teams

Doctors, nurses, and other professional disciplines are increasingly expected to carry out managerial functions and have responsibility for a team. Managers require a diverse range of skills and many feel threatened, especially in their first post. Often, people with professional backgrounds have superb clinical skills, but undeveloped managerial abilities. There are high costs if a team is not managed properly.

The manager

A manager should have good leadership potential. But the functions of a manager are more focused and specific than a leader. A manager will have:
- Clearly stated aims and objectives for their team – delegated to them by the wider organization.
- Authority to manage and order the working day of the team.
- Responsibility to ensure that the team complies with the wider organizational framework and regulation.

Management skills

In order to manage a team well, a manager will need to develop the following three groups of skills:
- *Communication* – clarity of vision and mission, clarity of expectation, fair, objective, and timely feedback, dissemination and liaison with the wider organization.
- *Leadership* – inclusion of team members, appropriate delegation, respect, motivation, and inspiration.
- *Organization* – time and people management, capacity management, quality assurance, budget management, project planning, and performance management.

Reasons why teams fail
- Lack of clearly defined aims and objectives for the team.
- Lack of clear management mandate.
- Poor understanding of the corporate context in which the team operates.
- Poor internal relationships.
- Poor supporting systems, procedures and processes, e.g. HR, IT, clinical protocols.
- Poor communication – both within the team and dissemination to and from the team within the wider organization.
- Poor levels of individual support, supervision, and development.
- Hindering behaviours and attitudes left unmanaged e.g. gossip, boredom, lack of engagement, dominance of a few people, lack of listening.
- Actions often taken prematurely prior to consultation, discussion, or planning.

Androulla Johnstone, Chief Executive, Health and Social Care Advisory Service

Reasons why teams succeed

- Clear goals and objectives that are clearly articulated and that are SMART (specific, measurable, achievable, realistic, and timed). These goals need to be established for the team and the individual in the annual appraisal process.
- Defined roles and functions clearly outlined in job descriptions and person specifications.
- Open and clear communication, including clarity of vision and expectation.
- Effective decision-making.
- Balanced participation recognizing the inputs of all team members, whilst acknowledging that the manager has the ultimate responsibility to decide upon the appropriate action required.
- Valued diversity.
- Managed conflict.
- Positive atmosphere.
- Effective systems and processes that provide a framework for effective functioning.

Further reading

French, WL, Bell, CH, Zawacki RA. *Organisational Development and Transformation: managing effective change.* McGraw Hill Publishing Co. London.
Makely, S Professionalism in health care. A Primer for carer success New Jersey. 2004.

Clinical supervision

Clinical supervision, regardless of professional affiliation, should be a mechanism for protecting standards and public safety, whilst supporting the development of excellence in practice. It is basically a space in which the dynamics of the working clinical world can be explored in a safe and confidential environment.

As well as there being a myriad of definitions, there is also a proliferation of models. Some common features of clinical supervision are listed below:

- It has a number of aims such as ensuring evidence based practice, skills development, professional growth, and personal support for the practitioner.
- The process requires formal structures and procedures to make it safe and effective.
- It is an active process requiring equal input from supervisee and supervisor.
- 📖 Practising in a reflective and professionally appropriate manner

Fundamentals of clinical supervision

Clinical supervision as a basic minimum should help to:
- Regulate standards.
- Develop professional function.
- Support the individual practitioner on a personal level.

Clinical supervision should not be confused with:
- **Appraisal** – this is a formal management process for the setting of job specific aims and objectives. It is primarily guided by the needs of the organization (📖 Personal development and appraisal).
- **Management supervision** – this is a formal process whereby a manager ensures that individuals who directly report to them are practicing effectively, achieving specific goals and targets, and are receiving regular feedback about their work-based performance (📖 Management supervision).
- **Counselling** – this is a formal therapeutic activity (📖 Counselling).
- **Mentoring** – this is an educational method whereby a student or learner is supported during a skills acquisition programme.
- **Caseload supervision** – this is a process that is primarily guided by the needs of the client or patient.

Clinical supervision differs from the activities listed above in that it is primarily structured and governed by the needs of the supervisee as an autonomous practising individual, seeking guidance and structured enquiry into their practice. Clinical supervision is not something that is 'done to' anyone. It is not a mandatory process. It is an 'adult' process for practitioners exploring the dynamics of the clinical world in which they work.

Androulla Johnstone, Chief Executive, Health and Social Care Advisory Service

Clinical supervision can be conducted in a variety of ways. The most common format is the one-to-one session or the group session. It is important that the clinical supervisor is not the manager of the supervisee and that, where possible, the supervisee should have some say as to who their supervisor is. The supervisee needs to be satisfied that the supervisor has the appropriate skills and experience to assist them at whatever stage they are at in their professional lives. All transactions should be entirely confidential, unless a breach of professional conduct is revealed during a clinical session. All issues regarding clinical supervision should be set down in a formal contract between the supervisor and the supervisee, with the basic ground rules being explained and agreed at the start of any supervision programme.

Further reading

Power, SC. *Nursing Supervision: a guide for clinical practice*. Sage Publications: London, 1999.
Scaife, J. *Supervision in the Mental Health Profession*. Taylor & Francis: 2001. London.

Management supervision

This is an active management mechanism to ensure that directly managed employees are working to agreed targets and processes with appropriate outcomes. It is an opportunity for reflection and feedback. Unlike clinical supervision, it is a directly managed process, where the employee's work is the focus of the meeting. The agenda should be shared between the supervising manager and the employee, but this is not a self-directed meeting for the employee, and the outcomes of such meetings are very much focused on performance management.

Kadushin defines management supervision as a process whereby the supervisor meets with a member of staff to whom they have delegated key responsibilities. This supervisory meeting acts to coordinate, enhance, and evaluate the performance of the supervisee for whose work they are held accountable.

📖 Practising in a reflective and professionally appropriate manner

Fundamentals of management supervision

Management supervision should:
- Have an agreed plan that includes the workplace aims and objectives of the supervisee.
- Include the provision of guidance, direction, feedback about performance and the identification of training and development needs.
- Be integral to the annual performance appraisal process.

It is quite likely that the direct line manager will perform management supervision. The supervisee will probably not have a choice in this matter. The process may feel challenging at times to all concerned, as the supervision will be based around the needs of the workplace and the ability of the supervisee to work in that environment.

Management supervision works best if the process is open, fair, and objective. Honest feedback is integral to the process. Some ground rules can help:
- Rarely, poor performance issues may be discussed that require formal human resource processes to be put into place. The supervisee needs to be aware that this is a course of action open to the supervisor.
- All supervisors must adhere to the human resource policies of their organization, bearing in mind dignity at work, disciplinary, and grievance policies. Shouting, bullying, and aggression are unacceptable behaviours.
- The supervision should be facilitative and developmental, ensuring that the supervisee accomplishes their workplace objectives.
- The supervisor should provide an opportunity for the supervisee to discuss any ideas they may have about improving their performance in the workplace.
- All transactions should take place in an adult and respectful manner.

Androulla Johnstone, Chief Executive, Health and Social Care Advisory Service

Further reading

Booyens, SW. *Introduction to Health Service Management*. Juta Accademic: 2004.
Hill, SS, Stephems, H. *Success in Practical/Vocational Nursing: from student to leader*.
   WB Saunders Company: 2001. Philedelphia

Personal development and appraisal

For an individual to perform well in the workplace, the organization needs to ensure that all employees:
- Understand clearly what is expected of them regarding workplace behavior, aims, and objectives.
- Know the key mission of their organization.
- Are practically equipped to do the job that they are employed to do- e.g. have access to a computer and a phone.
- Are trained and developed appropriately so that they can deliver their objectives.

The appraisal is usually an annual meeting between the employee and their manager, where a focused discussion takes place. The purpose is to identify the forthcoming annual aims and objectives for the individual, together with a developmental plan that will ensure successful support. The appraisal is usually supplemented by quarterly progress meetings and management supervision.

Fundamentals of appraisal

Appraisal is a formal developmental process of evaluation and structured discussion aimed at the personal, professional, and career development of the individual. Many organizations no longer combine this process with performance appraisal where the needs of the organisation are at the forefront of the discussion.

The appraisal should, as a minimum:
- Actively include the individual in the organization – it should explain the key organizational mission and goals, and help the individual understand how their role and department help the organization succeed.
- Explain the aims, objectives, and targets that have been set for the appraiser and the specific department in which they work.
- Negotiate with the appraisee about what their own contribution to the departmental aims and objectives will be.
- Identify the training and development needs of the individual if they are to achieve their goals for the year.
- Contain objectives that are SMART, i.e. specific, measurable, achievable, realistic, and timed.

The appraisal should not:
- Be regarded as an opportunity to suddenly cite the appraiser's concerns regarding the appraisees performance. This meeting should contain no surprises.
- Be sprung upon the appraisee without adequate preparation time. The appraisee should have access to all the necessary paperwork well in advance.
- Be hurried or carried out in an inappropriate venue e.g. phones should be diverted and do not disturb signs should be hung on doors.

Androulla Johnstone, Chief Executive, Health and Social Care Advisory Service

The personal development plan

Relevant training and development opportunities should be identified that support the appraisee and help them meet their aims and objectives. The opportunities identified should also consider the learning preferences of the appraisee. Training and development can be met in a variety of ways, for example:

- Coaching or clinical supervision.
- Directed reading.
- Shadowing a colleague inside or outside the organization.
- Short visits or secondments to another department or situation.
- Joining a working party or task force.
- Joining a learning set.
- Conferences.
- Short courses.
- Longer courses or continuing with academic studies.

NB Health and safety training must be included as mandatory each year.

Further reading

Grote, D. *Complete Guide to Performance Appraisal*. Amacon: 1996. New York.
Swan, WS. *How to do a Superior Performance Appraisal*. John Wiley & Sons: New Jersey 1991.

The effective acute psychiatric ward

An effective ward is one that:
- Keeps patients safe to the best possible degree.
- Accurately assesses the mental disorders and needs of each patient.
- Provides excellent care and treatment for mental and physical health.
- Assists, supports, and sometimes imposes self-care.
- Provides a respite location for patients, or by admitting a patient, provides respite to their relatives or carers.

The fact that these are the functions of acute wards, and the standards by which their efficacy should be judged, is shown by what staff say about their roles, and by the reasons for which patients are admitted.[5]

Running an effective ward is a whole team function. Although much of the day-to-day burden is carried by mental health nurses, it requires input from psychiatrists, occupational therapists, support workers, and others. A ward cannot be effective unless the whole multidisciplinary team works together in partnership with shared ideals and values.

Patient safety

Keeping patients safe means preventing them from harming themselves, others, and property. This sometimes requires coercion, for example, patients can be detained in hospital under the Mental Health Act (1983). Some argue that the best way to keep a patient safe is through the nurse-patient relationship, whereas others stress security policies and the use of containment, such as extra sedating medication or special observation. Both are required, but the most effective balance between them is subject to argument.

Factors that affect ward safety

Practice factors include:	*Service factors include:*
• Risk assessment and predication	• Ward design and ambience
• De-escalation techniques	• Social environment, case mix, forced cohabitation
• Observation	• Amount of time staff spend with patients
• Physical intervention (use of restraint)	• Leadership, morale, use of bank and agency staff
• Rapid tranquillization	
System factors:	*Population factors:*
Clinical, service and managerial systems that impact on ward safety.	The ward will reflect the qualities of the community from which its patients are drawn.

Professor Len Bowers, City University, London

Assessment

For an accurate assessment, nurses require a thorough knowledge of psychopathology, and the ability to observe patient behaviour and record or communicate those observations in a clear, succinct, and objective manner. If a patient's needs go unnoticed or uncommunicated, their treatment may be compromised.

Treatment

The provision of treatment by nurses should be done with care and attention to detail. Treatment is usually consensual; but due to the nature of mental disorder, it is occasionally legally coerced.

Self-care

Acute mental illness affects a person's ability to care for themselves, for example, to eat, drink, get enough sleep, stay clean, keep warm, and wear appropriate clothing. All these deficits need to be met and remedied by the effective nurse team working in partnership with patients.

References

5 Bowers, L, Clark, N, Callaghan, P. Multidisciplinary Reflections on Assessment for Compulsory Admission: The views of Approved Social Workers, General Practitioners, Ambulance Crews, Community Psychiatric Nurses and Psychiatrists. *British Journal of Social Work* **33**: 961–8, 2003.

Further reading

Department of Health. Mental Health Policy Implementation Guide: Acute In-patient care provision. DoH: London, 2002.
National Patient Safety Agency. Safer Wards in Acute Psychiatry. National Patient Safety Agency: London 2004.

The effective community mental health team

Introduction

The multidisciplinary team lies at the heart of modern health and social care. Collaboration between agencies and professional disciplines replaces divisions and demarcations, and improves the quality of service provision.

Types of teams

Community Mental Health Team (CMHT) – these are generic teams providing mental health care to the working age population of a geographical area. Similar teams operate for older people, referred to as CMHT Older People.

Assertive Outreach Teams – these are specialist teams providing assertive and intensive treatment to mentally ill people who frequently relapse and require inpatient treatment, or to those who are resistant to psychiatric treatment.

Home Treatment or Crisis Teams – these provide intensive care and support to people who would otherwise require admission to psychiatric hospital, or for vulnerable people who have been discharged from hospital.

Early Intervention Teams – these offer specialist treatment, information, and support to people experiencing their first psychotic illness.

Other specialist teams provide mental health services to members of black and ethnic minority communities, and to people who are homeless or who suffer from co-morbid substance misuse problems.

Effective teams

The effective care of severely mentally ill people requires a collaborative working relationship with the service user, and between psychiatrists, social workers, and mental health nurses. Optimal care requires the additional involvement of clinical psychologists, occupational therapists, support workers and increasingly, housing, welfare, and those who work with refugees or asylum seekers. Constructive partnerships, where appropriate, with primary care services and the family, are essential.

Multidisciplinary healthcare teams that work effectively produce better patient outcomes; including reduced mortality, greater continuity of care, and consistent communications with patients and families. They also develop shared knowledge and skills within the team.

Clear agreed aims, policies, and procedures are crucial. Teams with clear objectives, and higher levels of communication and member participation operate more effectively. Greater integration and respect for team members is associated with new and innovative ways of delivering patient care and improved mental well-being among staff.

Dr Alan Simpson, City University, London

Sufficient staff are required to provide a range of expertise and skills. Large teams can become overwhelmed by communication and line management difficulties.

Effective community mental health teams are associated with fewer suicides, greater continuity of care, shorter inpatient stays, less patient dissatisfaction, and lower costs.

Further reading

Onyett, S. *Team-working in mental health*. Palgrave: London, 2002.

Royal College of Psychiatrists. Community mental health care. Royal College of Psychiatrists: London, 2005. Available at: www.rcpsych.ac.uk/publications/cr/council/cr124.pdf

Promoting collaboration in primary mental health care

One in four people experience mental health problems of differing severity and complexity; and they require varying degrees of health and social support.

There is a growing interest in examining effective ways that people with mental health problems living in the community are provided with and can access safe, and responsive services. If the needs and aspirations of these people are not adequately addressed then they will continue to face social exclusion. It is important that all agencies, including central government, the NHS, local government, the independent sector, and providers of housing and employment schemes are aware of the issues and prepared to take action. The National Service Framework for Mental Health is clear about providing services that 'promote mental health for all'.[6]

📖 Health promotion
📖 Mental Health needs of the population

Why people with mental heath issues do not engage with services

The reasons for not using mental health services may include:

- Upbringing, life experiences, or attitudes.
- Feeling let down in the past.
- Stigma and discrimination.
- Negative staff attitudes e.g. racism or homophobia.
- Staff do not have the necessary skills.
- Purely biomedical approaches.
- No family or carer support.
- Lack of knowledge or information.

Services may not be able to effectively engage with individuals, families, and carers, due to factors such as prioritizing care, staff competencies, time, and resources.

What service users need

When service users were asked what they needed from services (The Sainsbury Centre for Mental Health), their replies included the following:

- Engagement.
- A range of treatments and care, including crisis intervention.
- An identified person, responsible 24 hours per day.
- A risk management approach, offering safety for the client and public.
- Consideration of social factors, as well as mental and medical issues.
- Supported access to mainstream services.
- Daytime activity – occupation, opportunity, and purpose.
- Help with finances and benefits.
- Suitable accommodation.

Dr Eddie McCann, City University, London

Recommendations for delivering effective and responsive health and social care

A government workforce team made several recommendations about what is needed to deliver effective health and social care that is responsive to the needs of people with mental health problems:[7]

- Skilled staff, including training and supervision.
- New roles e.g. graduate mental health workers, gateway workers.
- Needs-led services.
- Staff who are able to work in informal settings.
- Effective joint working for statutory and non-statutory sectors.
- A shared vision and common agenda.
- Developing positive staff attitudes in primary care.
- Focus on psychosocial interventions.
- Support for families and carers.
- Mental health awareness in schools, colleges, and the workplace.
- Assertive outreach, and a caseload ceiling of ten clients.
- More prison inreach staff.
- Community development workers for black and ethnic minorities.
- Outreach teams for personality disorder.

The overall aim is to develop a workforce with the competencies to give person-centred, socially inclusive, and recovery focused services in a multidisciplinary setting. To foster engagement, the person and their carers should be fully involved in decisions, given informed choices and treated with dignity and respect.

References

6 Department of Health. National Service Framework for Mental Health. HMSO: London, 1999.
7 Department of Health. Mental Health Care Group Workforce Team, National Mental Health Workforce Strategy. HMSO: London, 2004.

Further reading

The Sainsbury Centre for Mental Health. Keys to Engagement. SCMH: London, 1998.

Multi-agency working

Mental health nursing takes place in the context of work with other agencies also involved in the care of users. In this topic we will consider how mental health nurses can work effectively with other agencies.

📖 Planning and reviewing care programmes for people with mental health needs

Advantages of multi-agency working
- More efficient use of staff.
- Effective service provision.
- More satisfying work environment.
- More effective achievement of objectives.
- Seamless delivery of care.
- Less medicalization of mental health issues.
- Provides a medium for mental health awareness.
- Promotes an inclusive form of mental health care.

Working effectively with other agencies
In order to work effectively with other agencies, the mental health nurse needs to:
- Be capable of explaining their role and the parameters they work within.
- Be capable of communicating with other agencies.
- Understand the role and boundaries of other agencies.
- Be capable of engaging users in collaborative working across agencies through empowering and informing e.g. explaining the role of other agencies such as children and families social services.
- Recognize the part that significant others play in supporting the user.

Multi-agency teams
Mental health nurses will work with other agencies in the following teams:
- Community Mental Health Teams
- Assertive Outreach Teams
- Home Treatment or Crisis Teams
- Early Intervention Teams
- Other specialist teams e.g. those providing mental health services to members of black and ethnic minority communities, or to people who are homeless or suffer from co-morbid substance misuse problems.

It is also important to acknowledge the inter-agency capacity within the role of the acute in-patient nurse who will have to liaise and negotiate with other agencies such as the police, the Mental Health Act Commission and independent advocacy services as well as all the statutory authorities such as approved social workers (ASW).

Patrick Callaghan Professor of Mental Health Nursing, University of Nottingham & Nottinghamshire Healthcare NHS Trust

Health and social care organizations

Mental health nurses may work with the following health and social care organizations:
- Social services
- Benefits agency
- Groups involved in mental health care and support e.g. Mind, SANE, Rethink, Mental Health foundation
- Mental Health Act Commission
- Healthcare Commission
- Local authority housing departments and housing associations.

For cultural diversity, agencies such as:
- Jewish care
- Chinese mental health association

Further reading

Department of Health. The Ten Essential Shared Capabilities: A Framework for the Whole of the Mental Health Workforce. DoH: London, 2004.
Onyett, S. Team-working in mental health. Palgrave: London, 2002.

Working with advocacy services

Advocacy refers to the process of pleading the cause of and acting on behalf or another person, to secure services they need, and rights to which they are entitled. Advocates are independent of service providers and represent the interests of their advocacy partner as if they were their own.

Advocacy takes many shapes and forms, and provides both challenges and opportunities for nurses.

Self-advocacy

Self-advocacy is when individuals speaks out for themselves, and act on their own behalf. They might be supported by groups such as:

- *Self-help groups* – for people with particular diagnoses, or similar experiences e.g. groups of sexual abuse survivors, or people from minority ethnic communities.
- *Survivor groups* – campaigning independently, rather than working alongside service providers.
- *Advocacy projects and patients' councils* – working in a locality to support service users on hospital wards or in the community.
- *Service user forums* – local groups seeking changes, who participate in the planning, research, and evaluation of local mental health services, and provide training for mental health workers.

Some of these groups may not fall completely into one category, but may have several functions.

Group advocacy

Group advocacy is when groups are empowered to speak and be heard on specific issues, e.g. a patient's council, or a user group for a particular service. As well as being valuable sources of information and mutual support, these groups are able to give their opinions on services, lobby for new services or improvements to existing services. Advocacy groups can also decide to set up and run their own services, anything from social clubs to crisis houses.

Peer advocacy

This involves an individual being given the support of an advocate who has themselves used, or is using mental health services.

Legal advocacy

Legal advocacy is representation by legally qualified advocates, who are usually solicitors.
Some will specialize in clients detained under the Mental Health Act 1983.

Citizen advocacy

This is a long-term, one-to-one partnership, between a service user and an advocate who is a member of the public, usually as a part of a scheme coordinated by an organization or service.

Tina Coldham, National Development Consultant, Health and Social Care Advisory Service, London

Formal or professional advocacy

This term is often used for advocacy schemes that are staffed by paid professionals. They may be managed by large voluntary organizations. They sometimes adopt a so-called 'expert' model of advocacy, which involves giving advice, prioritizing options, counseling and mediation services.

Issues for nurses

When working with advocacy services nurses should:
- Adhere to any working agreements with the advocacy service.
- Respect the independence and principles of the advocacy service.
- Be aware of confidentiality issues – who tells whom what?
- Involve advocates in any health care meetings you hold with your clients.
- Adhere to employers sharing information policy.

Further reading

UK Advocacy Network: www.u-kan.co.uk
A Clear Voice, A Clear Vision: the advocacy reader. UKAN: 2001.
Advocacy – A Code of Practice. UKAN: 1994.
Advocacy Standard – Standards for advocacy in Mental Health. UKAN: 2004.
Advocacy Today and Tomorrow – The UK Advocacy Network Training Tool. UKAN: 2004.

Collaborative care

Collaborative care is the name for a systematic way of organizing the management of people with severe and enduring mental illness. It features close working relationships between primary care generalists such as GPs, and specialist mental health professionals, mediated through the introduction of a case manager into primary care.

Collaborative care has a very strong evidence base. More than 12,000 patients have been included in at least 34 randomized controlled trials of collaborative care. In trials, 70% of people with major depression achieve a 50% or more reduction in symptoms when treated in collaborative care systems, compared to 40% treated by usual care. It is effective in working with adults, older adults, and people with co-morbid physical conditions such as diabetes.

Elements of collaborative care

There are three elements of collaborative care:
1. Mechanisms to foster closer liaison between primary care clinicians and mental health specialists around individual patient care. These include regular meetings between primary care clinicians and specialists.
2. A case manager in primary care, to assist in the management of patients with depression through structured pharmacological and psychological interventions. Case managers provide patients with medication support and deliver low-intensity psychological interventions to patients.
3. Mechanisms to collect and share information on the progress of individual patients using shared information technology and primary care based notes.

Case management in collaborative care

Case management differs from traditional community mental health nursing practice. In collaborative care, case managers:
- Hold large volumes of active cases, typically 100 or more.
- Use the telephone as the most common form of contact with patients.
- Short contacts with patients, typically lasting no more than 10–20 minutes.
- Liaise with primary care clinicians around the care of individual patients.
- Receive regular scheduled caseload supervision from mental health specialists.
- Proactively contact depressed patients (often trying many times to contact them) identified by primary care clinicians.
- Integrate medication support with evidence-based low-intensity psychological treatments such as problem solving, self-help CBT or behavioural activation.
- 📖 Case management skills

Professor Dave Richards, University of York

Collaborative care is a complex and highly effective organizational strategy of quality improvement for depression management in primary care. Its combination of clinician education, consultation-liaison, and case management is underpinned by information systems and scheduled communications, enabling primary care to improve depression care significantly.

Further reading

Gilbody, S, Whitty, P, Grimshaw, J, et al. Educational and organizational interventions to improve the management of depression in primary care: a systematic review. *JAMA* **289**: 3145–51, 2003.

Unützer, J, Katon, W, Callahan, CM, et al. Collaborative care management of late life depression in the primary care setting: a randomized controlled trial. *JAMA* **288**: 2836–45, 2002.

Evidence-based mental health nursing

Introduction to evidence-based practice

Evidence-based practice is defined by Sackett *et al.* (1996, p. 71) as: 'the conscientious, explicit and judicious use of current best evidence in making decisions about the care of individual patients'.

What is evidence?

Evidence includes the following:
- The results of well-designed research studies especially those testing effectiveness like RCTs.
- Advice from experts endorsed by respected authorities.
- Clinical assessments of patients based on information gathered.
- Beliefs and values of practitioners.
- Patients' preferences.

Assessing the quality of evidence

Asking the following questions can help establish the quality of evidence:
- Is this the best type of research method for this question?
- Is the research of adequate quality?
- What is the size of the beneficial effect and of the adverse effect?
- Is it possible to generalize the research to the whole population from which the sample was drawn?
- Are the results applicable to the 'local' population?
- Are the results applicable to this patient?

The components of evidence-based practice

- The success or harm of all interventions.
- Clinical guidelines.
- Patient and public choice.
- Information on epidemiology.
- Evidence-based purchasing that reflects audit outcomes and performance measures.
- Health service management.
- Organizational audit.
- Financial audit and guidelines.
- Education and training.
- Curricula based on scientific evidence and research.

Skills required by the evidence-based mental health nurse

These skills include an ability to:
- Define criteria such as effectiveness, safety, and acceptability.
- Find articles on the effectiveness, safety and acceptability of a new test or treatment.
- Assess the quality of evidence.

Patrick Callaghan, Professor of Mental Health Nursing, University of Nottingham & Nottinghamshire Healthcare NHS Trust

- Assess whether the result of research can be generalized to the whole population from which the sample was drawn.
- Assess whether the results of the research are applicable to the 'local' population.

Critique of evidence-based practice

- The premise that health care should be based on the best available evidence is sound.
- Evidence-based practice is an authoritarian gesture with the purpose of bringing about conformity and compliance with questionable dogma.
- At what point is enough evidence gathered to justify a clinical decision?
- The integration of clinical acumen with current best evidence will improve competence and caring in health professionals.
- Health problems are not neatly resolved by recourse to research trials and hierarchies of evidence.
- Questions relating to the care of patients are not all answered by science.
- Health care is at the interface of many disciplines, not just epidemiology, as evidence-based practice seems to imply.
- The role of other types of evidence – such as that derived from qualitative research – have not been clearly delineated in evidence-based practice.

Best value: a complement to evidence-based practice?

Best value is a means of achieving improvements in social care that also has value for improving health care alongside evidence-based practice.

Factors for achieving best value in nursing

1. Ownership of problems and willingness to change.
2. A sustained focus on what matters.
3. The capacity and systems to deliver performance and improvement.
4. Integration of best value principles into all activities.

Principles for modernizing care using a best value approach

- Organizing services around people.
- Empowering people and supporting them to live their lives in the ways they choose.
- Step change approach to improving services so that users experience tangible changes.
- Recognizing the needs of carers.
- Delivering services in a seamless way.
- Ensuring services are sensitive to minority needs.
- Developing a confident and well-supported workforce.

Further reading

Gray, JAM. *Evidence-based Health Care*, Churchill-Livingstone: London, 1997.
Social Services Inspectorate/Audit Commission. Getting the best from best value: the experience of applying best value in social care. DoH: London, 2002.

Evaluating published evidence

The term evaluate means to judge the worth or value of something. Evaluation requires a balanced critique during which you will identify strengths and weaknesses of the published paper. Most research textbooks have a section on how to evaluate a published paper. The revised CONSORT statement[1] offers good guidance in critiquing randomized controlled trials. An excellent example is found in Polit and Beck[2] and a good example is Benton and Cormack.[3] Also, have look at the CASP (Critical Appraisal Skills Programme) website.[4] This website has 10 different checklists for critiquing 10 different types of research reports and is an indispensable source of useful information for critiquing research.

General tips on evaluating published research
- Be as objective as possible.
- Do not insult the author(s) or question their competence.
- Be reasonable in your critique.
- Give specific examples of the strengths and limitations of the paper.
- Be sensitive in making negative statements; put yourself in the authors' shoes.
- Try to justify your criticisms.
- Suggest alternatives.

The evaluation process
Most research reports are written using a particular structure with subsections describing each part of the research undertaken. You can use this structure to form your evaluation. In particular, your evaluation may focus on the following:
- Researchers' qualifications
- Title
- Abstract
- Introduction
- Background/literature review
- Theoretical/conceptual framework
- Research aims/questions/hypotheses (if any)
- Definition of key terms
- Research design
- Population and sample
- Data collection methods
- Data collection instruments (if any)
- Data analysis
- Discussion of findings
- Conclusions
- Implications
- Recommendations
- Overall impression.

Patrick Callaghan, Professor of Mental Health Nursing, University of Nottingham & Nottinghamshire Healthcare NHS Trust

Key Points

- It is important how you read, not just what you read.
- Being critical is a process, not an attitude.
- Use published criteria to help you review research papers.

References

1 Moher, D, Schulz, KF, Altman, DG. The CONSORT statement: revised recommendations for improving the quality of reports of parallel group randomized trials. *The Lancet* **357**: 1191–4, 2001.
2 Polit, DF, Beck, CT. *Nursing Research: Principles and Methods*, 7th edn. Lippincott: Philadelphia PA, 2004: pp..
3 Benton, DC, Cormack, DFS. Reviewing and evaluating the literature. In: DFS Cormack (ed.) *The Research Process in Nursing*, 4th edn. Blackwell Science: Oxford, 2000: pp..
4 Critical Appraisal Skills Programme website: www.phru.nhs.uk/CASP

Clinical governance

Clinical governance is central to the UK government's drive for quality improvements in the NHS. Clinical governance is the framework for delivering health services; and it is a method of helping services achieve the standards set out in the various National Service Frameworks. Clinical governance is the means to ensure local delivery of excellent care using the evidence provided by the National Institute of Health and Clinical Excellence (NICE). The Healthcare Commission monitors services to make sure the best available evidence is being used.

What is clinical governance?

Clinical governance is the method used by NHS organizations to deliver care and account for the quality of the care.

Features of clinical governance

Effective Leadership: where the vision, values, and methods of clinical governance are communicated to all staff.

Planning for quality: a plan to develop quality services is established based on an objective assessment of the needs and views of users, and exposure to risk. It identifies regulatory requirements, staff capabilities, unmet training needs, and an appreciation of how performance compares with best practice and similar services.

Being truly user-centered: this involves being clear about how feedback from users contributes to service planning and delivery.

Information, analysis, insight: this means having excellent systems for selecting, managing, and using information.

Good service design: this involves reflecting upon how services are designed, and changing services so that they are better designed to meet users' needs if necessary.

Demonstrating success: measures of quality and effectiveness are developed and used to demonstrate success.

Does clinical governance lead to better care?

The 2003 National Audit Office report is the first real evaluation of clinical governance. The main conclusions of this report are:
- Clinical governance has led to greater and more explicit accountability.
- It has also led to more open, transparent, and collaborative ways of working.
- The implementation of clinical governance is patchy across trusts.
- Trusts view clinical governance as having led to achievements in the structure and process of care delivery.
- The parts of clinical governance that meet statutory requirements without necessarily meeting the needs of patients are the most robust of all its components.

Patrick Callaghan, Professor of Mental Health Nursing, University of Nottingham & Nottinghamshire Healthcare NHS Trust

There is no direct evidence that improvements linked to clinical governance are directly improving patient care. There may be indirect improvements, as seen in the Healthcare Commission's Performance Ratings of Trusts, and in evidence from the National Patient Surveys.

Further reading

Nicholls, S, Cullen, R, O'Neill, S, et al. Clinical governance: its origins and its foundations. *Clinical Performance and Quality Health Care* **8**(3): 172–8, 2000.
The National Audit Office. Achieving Improvements through Clinical Governance. NAO: London, 2003.

Clinical audit

Clinical audit is a quality improvement process designed to improve care by evaluating the care against explicit criteria. Clinical audit is central to clinical governance.

Features of good clinical audit

- It should be part of a structured programme.
- Topics chosen for audit should be high risk, high volume, or high cost.
- Service should be part of the audit process.
- It should be multidisciplinary in nature.
- It should include assessment of the process and outcome of care.
- Standards should be derived from good quality guidelines.
- The sample size chosen should be adequate to produce credible outcomes.
- Managers should be directly involved in audit and any action plans arising from it.
- Action plans should address barriers to change, and identify those responsible for service improvement.
- Re-audit should be applied to ascertain whether improvements in care are as a result of clinical audit.
- Systems, structures, and specific mechanisms should be made available to monitor service improvements once the audit cycle is complete.
- Each audit should have a local lead.

The link between clinical audit and service improvement

Using clinical audit, service providers can examine whether:

- What ought to be happening is happening.
- Current practice meets required standards.
- Current practice follows published guidelines.
- Clinical practice is applying the knowledge that has been gained through research.
- Current evidence is being applied in a given situation.

There is no direct evidence that clinical audit leads directly to improvements in patient care. There may be indirect improvements as evidenced by Healthcare Commission Performance Ratings of Trusts and evidence from the National Patient Surveys. In the evaluation of clinical governance published by the National Audit Office in 2003,[5] clinical audit was perceived as extremely effective by one Trust, as very effective by 20 Trusts and as fairly effective by 61 Trusts. Seventeen Trusts reported clinical audit as not very effective and one Trust reported it as not at all effective.

Patrick Callaghan, Professor of Mental Health Nursing, University of Nottingham & Nottinghamshire Healthcare NHS Trust

Reference
5 The National Audit Office. Achieving Improvements through Clinical Governance. NAO: London, 2003.

Further reading
Clinical Governance Support Team. A Practical Handbook for Clinical Audit. DoH: London, 2005.
   Available at: www.cgsupport.nhs.uk/downloads/Practical_Clinical_Audit_Handbook_V1

Clinical guidelines

Clinical guidelines are systematically developed statements, which assist clinicians and patients in making decisions about appropriate treatment for specific conditions. The use of clinical guidelines is now widespread in many countries, and the evidence suggests that they do improve clinical practice, although the size of improvements varies greatly. Clinical guidelines are similar in many respects to care pathways and sometimes these terms are used synonymously.

Why clinical guidelines?
- They assist clinical decision-making by patients and practitioners.
- They educate individuals and groups.
- They assess and ensure the quality of care.
- They guide the allocation of resources.
- They reduce the risk of legal liability for negligent care.

Choosing an area to develop clinical guidelines
- Where there is excessive morbidity, disability, or mortality.
- Where treatment offers a good potential for reducing morbidity, disability, or mortality.
- Where there is wide variation in clinical practice.
- Where the services involved are resource intensive – either high volume and low cost, or low volume and high cost.
- Where there are many boundary issues involved, sometimes cutting across primary, secondary, and community care, and sometimes across different professional bodies.

Benefits and drawbacks of clinical guidelines

Benefits
- Holistic care.
- Greater inter-professional collaboration.
- Seamless package of care.
- Failure to achieve outcomes is quickly identified, as expected outcomes at different stages are specified.
- Can identify unmet needs.
- Should reduce treatment variation.
- Closer involvement of users.
- Care can be properly audited.
- Offer the best opportunity for effective and efficient care.
- Empower users.

Drawbacks
- May be rejected by clinicians because of constraints
- Initially developed in the USA to control costs
- They may restrict clinician's freedom

Patrick Callaghan, Professor of Mental Health Nursing, University of Nottingham & Nottinghamshire Healthcare NHS Trust

- Deviations from guidelines may be time consuming and costly
- Assumes that robust evidence exists – where it does not, there may not be agreement on most appropriate treatment.

Developing clinical guidelines

- Select topic
- Map current process
- Develop guideline
- Consult with providers and users
- Seek consensus
- Implement guideline
- Evaluate guideline
- Redesign if necessary.

Factors influencing the effectiveness of clinical guidelines

Relative probability of being effective	Development strategy	Dissemination strategy	Implementation strategy
High	Internal group	Specific educational intervention	Patient-specific reminder at time of consultation or treatment
Above average	Intermediate group	Continuing professional development	Patient-specific feedback
Below average	Local external group	Mailing to targeted groups	General feedback
Low	National external group	Publication in professional journal	General reminder of guideline

Further reading

Grimshaw, JM, Russell, IT. Effect of clinical guidelines on medical practice: a systematic review of rigorous evaluations. *The Lancet* **342**: 1317–22, 1993.
National Institute of Clinical Excellence. The Guideline Development Process: An overview for stakeholders, the public and the NHS. NICE: London, 2004.

The National Institute of Health and Clinical Excellence (NICE)

NICE[6] is responsible for providing national guidance on the promotion of good health and the prevention and treatment of ill health. NICE aims to combine knowledge and guidance on how to promote health and treat ill health.

What does NICE do?
NICE produces three main types of guidance on a range of health problems and issues:
- *Technology appraisals* – guidance on the use of new and existing medicines and treatments within the NHS in England and Wales.
- *Clinical guidelines* – guidance on the appropriate treatment and care of people with specific diseases and conditions within the NHS in England and Wales.
- *Interventional procedures* – guidance on whether interventional procedures used for diagnosis or treatment are safe enough and work well enough for routine use in England, Wales and Scotland.

The role of NICE in evidence-based health care
Within the NHS, NICE provides some of the evidence, and clinical governance is the means to ensure local delivery of excellent care using this evidence. The Healthcare Commission monitors services to make sure that the best available evidence is being used.

Patrick Callaghan, Professor of Mental Health Nursing, University of Nottingham & Nottinghamshire Healthcare NHS Trust

Reference

6 National Institute of Clinical Excellence website: www.nice.org.uk

The Healthcare Commission

The Healthcare Commission[7] is the independent inspection body for the NHS and the independent health care sector.

The role of the Healthcare Commission

Inspect
To inspect the quality and value for money of health care and public health services.

Inform
To equip patients and the public with the best possible information about the provision of health care.

Improve
To promote improvements in health care and public health.

The statutory duties of the Healthcare Commission
- To assess the management, provision, and quality of NHS health care and public health services.
- To review the performance of each NHS trust and to award them an annual performance rating.
- To regulate the independent health care sector through registration, annual inspection, monitoring complaints, and enforcement.
- To publish information about the state of health care.
- To consider complaints about NHS organizations that the organizations themselves have not resolved.
- To promote the coordination of reviews and assessments carried out by the commission and others.
- To carry out investigations of serious failures in the provision of healthcare.

In carrying out its duties, the Healthcare Commission pays particular attention to:
- The availability of, access to, and the quality and effectiveness of health care.
- The economy and efficiency of the provision of health care.
- The availability of and the quality of information provided to the public about health care.
- The need to safeguard and promote the rights and welfare of children and the effectiveness of such measures.

How the Healthcare Commission works
The Healthcare Commission is responsible for assessing and publishing information on the performance of NHS and independent health care services through:
- Annual health checks
- Performance ratings. Reviews and inspections
- Standards to assess performance.

Patrick Callaghan, Professor of Mental Health Nursing, University of Nottingham & Nottinghamshire Healthcare NHS Trust

The strategic goals of the Healthcare Commission

- *To promote a better experience of health and healthcare for patients and the public* – through fair and credible systems for assessing and rating performance across the NHS and the independent sector.
- *To safeguard the public* – by acting swiftly and appropriately on complaints, concerns, and significant failings in the provision of health care.
- *To provide authoritative, independent, relevant, and accessible information* – about what is going on in health care and the opportunities for improvement.
- *To promote action to reduce inequalities in people's health* - to improve their experiences of health care and access to services through greater respect for human rights and diversity.
- *To take a lead in coordinating and improving the impact and value for money of assessment and regulation in health care.*
- *To support their staff in creating an efficient, flexible, and highly skilled organization* – delivering world class assessment and regulation.

Reference

7 The Healthcare Commission website: www.healthcarecommission.org.uk

Disseminating and implementing evidence to improve practice

The overall aim of systematic reviews and clinical guidelines is to improve the quality of health care, and in the long-term to improve health outcomes. However, this will only happen if the evidence generated by reviews gets into policy and practice. Clinical guidelines are one way of getting evidence into practice. Described below are different methods of dissemination and implementation that have been shown to be effective in getting evidence into practice.

Definitions
Dissemination: the process through which target groups become aware of, receive, accept, and utilize information.
Diffusion: a passive process by which information is spread to an audience.
Implementation: activities aimed at improving the compliance of the target group with the recommendations about changes in clinical practice and health policy.

What works? Evidence-based methods of effective dissemination and implementation
- Academic detailing – providing lectures
- Opinion leaders – people who are regarded as influential and credible
- Audit/feedback
- Reminder systems
- Patient mediated interventions.

Consistently effective interventions
- Educational outreach visits
- Reminders
- Multifaceted interventions (e.g. two or more of audit and feedback reminders, local consensus processes, marketing)
- Interactive educational meetings.

Interventions of variable effectiveness
- Audit and feedback
- Local opinion leaders
- Local consensus processes
- Patient-mediated interventions.

Interventions that have little or no effect
- Educational materials
- Didactic educational meetings.

Patrick Callaghan, Professor of Mental Health Nursing, University of Nottingham & Nottinghamshire Healthcare NHS Trust

Putting evidence into practice: a report from 15 projects funded by the London Regional Office of the NHS ME

Factors related to likelihood of success

- Sufficient resources (e.g. time. money, and skills).
- Proposed change needs to offer benefits to front-line staff.
- Enough of the right people need to be on board early enough.
- Interactive approach linking research clearly to practice.

Key lessons of the project

- Expect to take several years.
- Successful implementation requires pragmatism and flexibility.
- Start small and build incrementally.
- Use what is already there.
- Target enthusiasts first.

Outcomes of the project

- Better relationships.
- Improved knowledge, systems, and skills.
- Practice change.
- Improved patent care.

Further reading

Bero, LA, Grilli, R, Grimshaw, JM, et al. Closing the gap between research and practice: an overview of systematic reviews of interventions to promote the implementation of research findings. *British Medical Journal* **317**: 465–8, 1997.

Wye, L, McClenahan, J. *Getting better with evidence: experiences of putting evidence into practice.* King's Fund: London, 2000.

Systematic reviews

A systematic review is a review of the evidence on a clearly formulated question. It uses systematic and explicit methods to identify, select, and critically appraise relevant primary research and to extract and analyse data from the studies that are included in the review. Statistical methods (meta-analysis) may or may not be used.

Strengths of systematic reviews

- They give comprehensive coverage – they may include studies using various research methods.
- Large amounts of information can be summarized concisely.
- Data from previous studies can be re-analysed, to present a composite picture.
- They are a useful aid in practitioners' pursuit of evidence-based health care.
- They can assist in the formation of effective social and health policy.
- They provide information on how effective an intervention is.
- They reduce the need for guesswork on the part of readers.

Weaknesses of systematic reviews

- There may be subjectivity in data inclusion, analysis, and reporting in that ultimately what gets included is decided by the reviewers.
- Coverage of the topic is restricted by the specific inclusion criteria.
- The effects of an intervention could be explained by many variables, not just the ones reported.
- Data from the studies may not be homogeneous.
- The studies may be combined inappropriately in that studies using different methods or different participants may be analysed together.

Steps in the systematic review process

- Identification of the need for a review
- Background research and problem specification
- Drawing up the requirements for the review protocol
- Literature searching and retrieval
- Judging studies for inclusion
- Assessing the validity of studies
- Data extraction
- Data synthesis
- Report.

Methods of identifying evidence for inclusion in systematic reviews

- Database searching
- Hand searching
- Searching reference lists of identified studies
- Contacting researchers in the field
- Finding unpublished literature.

Patrick Callaghan, Professor of Mental Health Nursing, University of Nottingham & Nottinghamshire Healthcare NHS Trust

Evaluating the quality of systematic reviews
The following questions might help you evaluate a systematic review:
- Does the review answer a well-defined question?
- Has there been a substantial effort to search for all the available literature (including unpublished literature)?
- Are the inclusion/exclusion criteria reported and appropriate?
- Is the validity of included studies adequately addressed?
- Are the individual studies presented in sufficient detail?
- Have the primary studies been combined or summarised appropriately?
- How sensitive are the results to changes in the way the review is done?
- Are judgments about preferences explicit?
- Are sub-group analyses interpreted cautiously?
- If there is 'no evidence of effect', is caution taken not to interpret this as 'evidence of no effect'?

The role of systematic reviews in evidence-based mental health nursing
- They are an important source of information for the development of clinical guidelines/best practice sheets.
- They are an efficient scientific technique.
- They can save professionals considerable time in accessing information.
- They can save money.

Further reading
Centre for Reviews and Dissemination, University of York. Undertaking Systematic Reviews of Research on Effectiveness. *CRD Report 4*, 2nd edn. University of York: York, 2001.
Greenhalgh, T, Donald, A. *Evidence Based Health Care Workbook For Individual and Group Learning.* BMJ Books: London, 2000.

Research

The research process

Research is the process of generating new knowledge through systematic enquiry governed by scientific principles.

Why do research?

- Improve practice.
- Defend practice.
- Increase body of knowledge.
- Widen repertoire of interventions.
- Improve cost-effectiveness.
- Provide evidence to support demands for extra resources.
- Satisfy academic or intellectual curiosity.
- Facilitate inter-professional collaboration.
- Earn and defend a professional status.

The research process

- Setting research questions(s), objectives, and (where appropriate) hypotheses.
- Searching and retrieving literature.
- Reviewing literature.
- Preparing a research proposal.
- Gaining ethical approval.
- Accessing research site.
- Collecting data.
- Handling and/or processing collected data.
- Disseminating, diffusing, and implementing research results.

The five phases of research

Conceptual phase

This phase involves formulating the research problem, reviewing related literature, defining a theoretical framework, and formulating hypotheses, research questions, or objectives.

Design and planning

This involves selecting the research design, identifying the sampling frame and the research sample, specifying methods, finalizing the research plan, obtaining ethical approval, conducting the pilot study, and making revisions to the original proposal if necessary.

Empirical

During this phase you will collect data and prepare the data for analysis.

Analytical

This phase is involves analysing the data and interpreting the results.

Dissemination

In this phase you will communicate and implement the findings of the research through evidence-based activities such as educational outreach visits and interactive educational meetings.

Patrick Callaghan, Professor of Mental Health Nursing, University of Nottingham & Nottinghamshire Healthcare NHS Trust

Uses of research in mental health nursing
- Practice
- Education
- Service development
- Management
- Policy

Further reading

Polit, DF., Beck, C. *Nursing Research, Principles and Methods*, 6th edn. Lippincott: Philadelphia PA, 2004.

Robson, C. *Real World Research*, 2nd edn. Blackwell: Oxford, 2001.

Philosophical assumptions underlying quantitative research

Quantitative approaches are used when researchers wish to test theory, other assumptions, and relationships between two or more variables. The quantitative research process usually follows predetermined stages.

Empiricism

Often called 'British empiricism' after the work of British philosophers: Berkeley, Hume, and Locke. Empiricism holds that knowledge derived from experience is more scientific; it provides better evidence as opposed to knowledge that derives from the senses or by the use of reason.

Assumptions of empiricism
- We should be sceptical about conclusions reached by the use of reason or the senses.
- Scrupulous (empirical) observation of human life allows us to develop laws about human behaviour.

Critique of empiricism
- It has led to more use of scientific methods to generate data.
- It has promoted the development of experimental methods in the health, human, and behavioural sciences.
- It undermines the role of reasoning, which may be useful in generating ideas to be tested empirically.
- Reason is necessary to understand the meaning and application of knowledge generated empirically.

Logical positivism

Also called logical empiricism, positivism originates from the work of a group of philosophers – known as the Vienna Circle – in the 1920s. Empiricism holds that knowledge derives from personal experience. Positivism holds that knowledge ultimately rests upon public experimental verification.

Assumptions of positivism
- Metaphysical rules are meaningless.
- All genuine knowledge can be expressed in a single language, common to all sciences.
- Theories that cannot be tested are not scientific.
- The aim of science is to seek causality, not meaning.
- A theory is scientific only if it generates universal knowledge.
- There is an objective reality than can be studied, measured, and understood.

Patrick Callaghan, Professor of Mental Health Nursing, University of Nottingham & Nottinghamshire Healthcare NHS Trust

Critique of positivism

- Reductionist (or focused?).
- Narrow view of science.
- Few theories can generate universal knowledge.
- The application of positivism has led to significant (health) discoveries.
- Human behaviour involves meaningful intentions, expectations, and action.
- Different sciences have different languages – the language of social sciences differs from that of natural sciences.
- Reality can only be approximated, not fully understood.
- Has generated universal theories.

Falsificationism

Falsificationism derived from the work of Karl Popper first published in 1935 (in German; 1959 in English).[1]

- Theories derive from deductive testing of ideas.
- Refutability is at the heart of scientific reasoning.
- Falsification (proving something to be false), not verification, is crucial in science.

Critique of falsificationism

- Theories can never be truly established.
- Theory acceptance is tentative, theory rejection can be decisive.
- Some well-established theories may have been rejected at birth.

The relationship of empiricism, positivism, and falsificationism to health and social care research

Arguably, logical positivism no longer exists in its purest forms. Contemporary empiricism is more suited to health and social care research. It is characterized by identifying factors thought to be the key to understanding and explaining health and social phenomena, theory testing and generation.

Contemporary empiricism, positivism, and falsificationism may be reflected in mental health nursing research by:

- Research methods; including experimental designs, observations, correlational designs.
- Developing empirical indicators of human behaviour.
- Theory development and testing.
- Building and strengthening the professional status of nursing.

- Summary of core differences between quantitative and qualitative research approaches

Criteria	Quantitative	Qualitative
Use of positivism	Modified: contemporary empiricism	No
Acceptance of postmodern ideas	Not likely: PM may be seen as an attack on reason and truth	Increasing use
Capturing the individual's point of view	Yes, through reliable, objective measures	Yes, through detailed observation and interviewing
Examining the constraints of everyday life	Yes, through 'etic' perspectives based on probabilities derived from large data sets selected at random	Yes, through direct confrontation: the 'emic' perspective
Securing 'rich' descriptions	Less important	Valuable

Conclusion

Researchers often treat quantitative and qualitative approaches as competing opposites in the battle for the supremacy of ideas and knowledge. The reality is that there are many sources of knowledge and each has the potential to inform those with an open and critical mind.

Reference

1 Popper, K. *The Logic of Scientific Discovery*, UK edn. Routledge: London, 1959.

Further reading

Gortner, SR. Nursing's syntax revisited: a critique of philosophies said to influence nursing theories. *International Journal of Nursing Studies* **30**(6): 477–88, 1993.

Qualitative approaches to research

When researchers use qualitative approaches they are usually collecting or analysing narrative data (words), in order to understand a social setting or phenomena, without preconceived notions of what they may find.

Qualitative research designs

Ethnography: investigating meanings, patterns, and experiences in defined cultural groups.

Phenomenology: exploring the lived experience or real world experience of individuals.

Ethology: investigating people's behaviour in a natural setting.

Grounded theory: investigating social processes within a defined social setting.

Symbolic interaction: studying the way in which people interact in social groups and the sense people make of these settings.

Discourse analysis: investigating the nature of written and verbal dialogue.

Assessing quality in qualitative research approaches

Credibility is a term used in qualitative research to demonstrate the reliability, validity, and quality of research methods. It differs in many respects to the notion of reliability and the validity methods used in quantitative research.

Improving credibility in qualitative research

- Respondent validation or member checking.
- Triangulation of methods, data, investigators, and theories.
- Clear exposition of data collection methods.
- Clear exposition of the process of data analysis.
- Reflexivity – examining the role of the researcher in the outcomes.
- Attention to negative cases; avoiding holistic bias.

Patrick Callaghan, Professor of Mental Health Nursing, University of Nottingham & Nottinghamshire Healthcare NHS Trust

Comparing qualitative and quantitative approaches to research

Criteria	Quantitative	Qualitative
Use of positivism	Modified: contemporary empiricism	No
Acceptance of postmodern ideas	Not likely: PM may be seen as an attack on reason and truth	Increasing use
Capturing the individual's point of view	Yes, through reliable, objective measures	Yes, through detailed observation and interviewing
Examining the constraints of everyday life	Yes, through 'etic' perspectives based on probabilities derived from large data sets selected at random	Yes, through direct confrontation: the 'emic' perspective
Securing 'rich' descriptions	Less important	Valuable

Further reading

Denzin, NK, Lincoln, YS (eds.). *Handbook of Qualitative Research*, 2nd edn. Sage: Thousand Oaks, CA, 2000.

Forming research questions

The research process often begins with the development of research questions. This usually happens during the conceptual stage of the research process (see 🔲 Forming research questions for a description of this stage).

Sources of research questions

Experience

Researchers will often have experience of the topic they are interested in and they may draw upon this experience to find research questions.

Social issues

These are a useful source of research questions. Researchers will often consider a range of social issues; especially those that indicate significant social problems or concerns. For example, increases in antisocial behaviour by young people may be considered a significant social issue, and research might help to understand the nature and causes of such behaviour.

Public health issues

These are issues that are often of concern to public health. For example, the increases in MRSA infection among people admitted to hospital or the rise of tuberculosis.

Policy issues

These are issues that arise from government policies. For example, the National Service Framework for Mental Health provides a rich source of potential research questions.

Theory

Nursing, health, and social care theories, or theories of human behaviour are rich sources of research questions. For example, Peplau[2] argues that mental health nursing is an interpersonal process in which the nurse plays various roles: resource person, surrogate parent, and leader. Research questions arising from this theory could investigate whether Peplau's views can be substantiated by research or applied across all areas of mental health nursing.

External sources

These include ideas suggested by others; they may be colleagues or experts in the field of interest or users of services.

Developing and refining a research problem

- Select the problem
- Narrow the problem
- Evaluate the problem

Evaluating a research problem

- What is the significance of the problem?
- How researchable is the problem?
- How feasible is it to address the problem?

Patrick Callaghan, Professor of Mental Health Nursing, University of Nottingham & Nottinghamshire Healthcare NHS Trust

Assessing the feasibility of research problems

- Time and timing
- Availability of study participants
- Cooperation of others
- Facilities and equipment
- Money
- Experience of researcher(s)
- Ethical considerations

Examples of research problems and research questions

Problem	Research question
Unsure how young people experience mental health difficulties.	How do young people experience mental health difficulties?
Limited evidence about how ward rules and regulations impact upon patients in acute psychiatric wards.	What is the impact of ward rules and regulations on patients in acute psychiatric wards?
Lack of understanding about whether cognitive behaviour therapy (CBT) is better than Interpersonal Psychotherapy (IPT) in helping people cope with depression.	How does CBT compare with IPT in helping people cope with depression?

Reference

2 Peplau, H. Interpersonal Relations in Nursing, a conceptual framework for psychodynamic nursing. New York: Putan 1952.

Further reading

Polit, DF, Beck, C. *Nursing Research, Principles and Methods*, 6th edn. Lippincott: Philadelphia PA, 2004.

Robson, C. *Real World Research*, 2nd edn. Blackwell: Oxford, 2001.

Research designs

A research design is a description of the specific research approach employed by researchers. There are a variety of research designs; the choice of design depends largely on the research questions. Below are examples of commonly used research designs.

Quantitative research designs

Randomized controlled trial (RCT) (also known as experimental design)

Often called the gold standard of quantitative designs, the RCT is used to test cause and effect relationships between at least two variables.

Survey

This involves collecting data in the form of questionnaires sent by post, structured face-to-face interviews, or telephone interviews.

Single case study

This is a highly structured study of one person.

Comparative

This involves the comparison of at least two nominal groups.

Factorial

This design involves the researcher studying the relationship between multiple variables.

Qualitative research designs

Ethnography

This is the study of people in their natural setting, through observation and interviews.

Phenomenology

This is study of the lived experience, or real world experience of individuals, by means of unstructured or semi-structured interviews.

Action research

This involves the study of health and social care systems with a view to addressing identified problems. A researcher doing action research will work in collaboration with people inside the systems they are studying, using a variety of research methods.

There are other research designs, for example, historical research, symbolic interaction, or longitudinal. Some are only used within one research tradition and others straddle both research traditions.

Triangulated designs involve the use of two or more methods in the same study.

Patrick Callaghan, Professor of Mental Health Nursing, University of Nottingham & Nottinghamshire Healthcare NHS Trust

Further reading

Bowling, A. *Research Methods in Health*, 2nd edn. Open University Press: Buckingham, 2002.

Denzin, NK, Lincoln, YS (eds.). *Handbook of Qualitative Research*, 2nd edn. Sage: Thousand Oaks, CA, 2000.

Well-designed quantitative studies

The ultimate quality of quantitative research depends on the extent that it minimizes threats to validity. 'Good' quantitative research designs are those that are appropriate to the research question and to the aims and objectives of the research, lack bias, are precise, and have an appropriate statistical power.

Categories of quantitative research designs
- Cross-sectional
- Longitudinal
- Comparative
- Retrospective
- Prospective.

Types of quantitative research designs
- Experimental
- Quasi-experimental
- Solomon 4 group – essentially where you have 2 experimental and 2 control groups
- Factorial
- Repeated measures
- Randomized controlled trials
- Time series
- Single case
- Correlational
- Case study
- Evaluation
- Survey
- Delphi
- Secondary analysis
- Meta-analysis
- Methodological.

Threats to internal and external validity
Internal validity occurs when the outcomes result only from the effect of the independent variable. Threats to internal validity arise from:
- Lack of control of 'noise'
- The history of the subjects
- Sample selection
- Maturation of subjects
- Effects of previous testing
- Bias in research instruments
- Response bias
- Lack of adequate statistical power
- Attrition or mortality – this is when participants withdraw from the study
- Setting significance level too high.

Patrick Callaghan, Professor of Mental Health Nursing, University of Nottingham & Nottinghamshire Healthcare NHS Trust

Dealing with threats to internal validity
- Better design
- Homogeneity
- Use of reliable and valid measures
- Increasing the size of the population sampled.

External validity is the potential of the research to generalise to other situations. Threats to external validity include:
- The Hawthorne Effect – where participants respond simply because of the attention they get from the researcher.
- Unrepresentative samples (number and quality).
- The novelty of new experiences for researchers and subjects alike.
- Characteristics of the researcher.
- Measurement effects – changes occurring from simple exposure to the data collection methods.

Dealing with threats to external validity
- Standard protocols
- Double blind procedures
- Supervision
- Having an adequate sample that will allow detection of changes predicted with confidence
- Having a representative sample.

Controlling for 'noise'
In quantitative research design it is important to control the variables that might have a causal or related effect on your research outcomes. This is known as 'noise'. Ways of controlling 'noise' include:
- Randomization
- Repeated measures
- Homogeneity
- Blocking
- Matching
- ANCOVA (Analysis of Covariance)

Note: Measures to improve the internal validity of a study often unavoidably interfere with external validity. This may have to be accepted as internal validity is more important.

Further reading
Polit, DF, Beck, C. *Nursing Research, Principles and Methods*, 6th edn. Lippincott: Philadelphia PA, 2004.
Robson, C. *Real World Research*, 2nd edn. Blackwell: Oxford, 2001.

Sampling

What is sampling?

Sampling is the process of deciding on the number and characteristics of the people who will be invited to participate in a study. Sampling is a process of selecting part of a population to represent the entire population. However, because the researcher may want to make comments about the entire population from their sample, it must be representative of the entire population.

There are two broad approaches to sampling:

Probability sampling – where the researcher uses *random sampling* to select respondents.

Non-probability sampling – where the researcher uses *non-random sampling*.

Probability sampling

Simple random sampling

Every member of the entire population has an equal chance of being selected. Firstly, the entire, eligible population – **the sampling frame** – is identified. Then the researcher randomly selects from this population by using random numbers, or pulling names out of a hat or card index for example. Simple random sampling may mean the sample is not representative.

Stratified random sampling

The researcher first divides the population into different groups, or strata. Then, a sample is randomly selected from each group, making the sample more representative of the entire population.

Cluster random sampling

This involves reducing large groups into small clusters (groups of similar things), and randomly selecting from within these clusters. This type of sampling is used to reduce the demands of surveying large groups, which might be time consuming, expensive, and unnecessary.

Systematic random sampling

This involves selecting every nth person from a list or group. For example if you need a sample size of 150 from a sampling frame of 40,000, divide 40,000 by 150 and you get 266. Every 266th person from your sampling frame would be selected until you reached 150.

Non-probability sampling

Convenience sampling

This uses the most conveniently available group of people. It is sometimes called opportunistic sampling, and may be used when it is not possible to use random sampling, or to save time. The use of convenience sampling is not likely to lead to a representative sample.

Patrick Callaghan, Professor of Mental Health Nursing, University of Nottingham & Nottinghamshire Healthcare NHS Trust

Quota sampling

This involves sampling different groups, but not randomly. It is basically a combination of purposive and stratified sampling, but without random selection.

Purposive sampling

This is sometimes called judgmental sampling or theoretical sampling. The researcher uses his or her knowledge of the sample to select who should be included in the study. The sample is selected because it is felt they might be typical of the sampling frame.

Snowball sampling

In this sampling method, respondents refer someone they know to the researcher. The sample is selected on the basis of the researcher collecting contacts from respondents incrementally (the snowball effect).

Important issues to consider in sampling

- Inclusion and exclusion criteria
- Sample size
- Attrition – where participants withdraw from the study
- Bias – in responses and sampling methods

Steps in the sampling process

- Identify the target population
- Identify the accessible population
- Specify eligibility criteria
- Specify sampling plan
- Recruit sample

Further reading

Cormack, DFS (ed.). *The Research Process in Nursing*, 4th edn. Blackwell Science: Oxford, 2000.
Polit, DF, Beck, C. *Nursing Research, Principles and Methods*, 6th edn. Lippincott: Philadelphia PA, 2004.

Qualitative methods of data collection

Observations and interviews are the most common data collection methods used in mental health nursing research. These methods are preferred because they allow a greater insight into a person's experience and the meaning they attach to that experience.

Observational methods

This method involves the systematic selection, observation, and recording of behaviour, events, and settings relevant to a research problem. Observations may be structured, or unstructured. The former are more likely in quantitative studies.

What is observed?
- Characteristics and conditions of individuals
- Verbal and non-verbal behaviours
- Activities
- Skill attainment and performance
- Environmental characteristics

Strengths of observational methods
- Comprehensive
- More natural setting
- May validate other methods
- Provides 'richer' data

Weaknesses of observational methods
- Observer bias and influence
- Creates artificial setting
- Intrusive
- Labour intensive
- Training required
- Costly

Strengths of interviews
- Provide high response rates
- May be more acceptable to participants
- Allow opportunities to improve clarity
- Allow a more in-depth discussion
- Participants less likely to miss questions
- Order of questions can be controlled
- Greater control over participant – you know who has provided data
- Supplementary data can be produced more readily

Patrick Callaghan , Professor of Mental Health Nursing, University of Nottingham & Nottinghamshire Healthcare NHS Trust

Weaknesses of interviews
- Costly and time consuming
- Lack of anonymity
- Interviewer bias
- Participants have less control
- Involves the use of expensive equipment such as tape recorders or MP3 players
- More intrusive in that the researcher has an opportunity to probe more deeply into issues which may be less possible with other methods such as questionnaires
- Not always as acceptable to participants
- Possibility of response bias.

Further reading

Denzin, NK, Lincoln, YS (eds.). *Handbook of Qualitative Research*, 2nd edn. Sage: Thousand Oaks, CA, 2000.

Qualitative data analysis

The analysis of qualitative data requires clear thinking and attention to detail on the part of the analyst. In qualitative data analysis the researcher is like a research tool; there is a great need for reflection, sensitivity, awareness, and/or bracketing (setting aside) of biases. There are many approaches to analysis, but there are features that most approaches have in common.

The focus of qualitative analysis

The focus of qualitative analysis is on:
- The characteristics of language
- The discovery of regularities
- The comprehension of the meaning of text
- Reflection.

Types of qualitative data analysis

Quasi-statistical methods: involves the use of statistical procedures, such as counting how often forms of narrative data occur. Content analysis is an example of a quasi-statistical method.

Template approaches: themes and codes may be predetermined prior to the analysis and a template developed. The researcher then searches the data for evidence of these themes and codes. Matrix analysis is an example of a template approach.

Editing approaches: involve no predetermined themes and codes, only those based on the researcher's interpretation of the text. Grounded theory is an example of an editing approach.

Immersion approaches: this approach is close to artistic interpretation, with little structure.

Common features of qualitative data analysis

- Coding data
- Adding comments
- Identifying themes, categories, sequences, relationships, and differences between groups
- Checking these themes with participants
- Generating a small set of generalized themes describing the consistencies from the analysis
- Linking these generalized themes to theories.

Patrick Callaghan, Professor of Mental Health Nursing, University of Nottingham & Nottinghamshire Healthcare NHS Trust

Further reading

Miles, MB, Huberman, AM. *Qualitative Data Analysis*, 2nd edn. Beverly Hills, Sage Publications 1994.

Robson, C. *Real World Research*, 2nd edn. Blackwell: Oxford, 2001.

Quantitative methods of data collection

Questionnaires, observations, and interviews are the most common data collection methods in mental health nursing research. Questionnaires are popular because they are easy to use and can collect research data from large samples, spread over a wide geographical area. Researchers may design a questionnaire, modify a questionnaire designed by others, or use a questionnaire designed by others without amendment. Observation and interviews are often used because they allow a greater insight into a person's experience, and the meaning they attach to that experience.

Questionnaires (e.g. Likert scales)
Strengths of questionnaires
- Relatively cheap
- Easy to use
- Less time consuming for both researcher and subject
- Allow subjects to reply at their own convenience
- Gives subjects control – they can check their responses for accuracy
- Greater confidentiality and anonymity for subjects
- Avoids interviewer bias
- Allows easier and faster data analysis
- Reliable – subjects are asked the same questions
- Researcher does not have to rely on memory, tape recorders, or note-taking.

Limitations of questionnaires
- Respondents may be dishonest
- Social desirability bias
- Subjects' responses may be restricted
- Reveal little about context in which responses were formed
- Cannot be certain that the person sent the questionnaire is the respondent
- Respondents may gauge researcher's intention and respond accordingly
- High risk of non-responses.

A serious weakness of questionnaires is the risk of a low response rate. The following may help improve your response rate:
- Estimating response rate and making necessary allowances
- Warn potential subjects in advance
- Explain how subjects were selected
- Sponsorship
- Personalize envelope
- Publicize study
- Offer incentives
- Assure confidentiality
- Issue reminders
- Ensure anonymity

Patrick Callaghan, Professor of Mental Health Nursing, University of Nottingham & Nottinghamshire Healthcare NHS Trust

- Enhance appearance of questionnaire
- Shorten length if possible
- Provide return envelopes
- Highlight the interest of the topic to the subject
- Build rapport with participants.

Observational methods

This involves the systematic selection, observation, and recording of behaviour, events, and settings relevant to a research problem. Observations may structured or unstructured. The former are more likely in quantitative studies.

What is observed?

- Characteristics and conditions of individuals
- Verbal and non-verbal behaviours
- Activities
- Skill attainment and performance
- Environmental characteristics.

Strengths of observational methods

- Comprehensive
- More natural setting
- May validate other methods
- Provides 'richer' data

Weaknesses of observational methods

- Observer bias and influence
- Creates an artificial setting
- Intrusive
- Labour intensive
- Training required
- Costly.

Structured interviews

Strengths of structured interviews

- High response rates
- May be more acceptable to participants
- Allow opportunities to improve clarity
- Allow a more in-depth discussion
- Participants less likely to miss questions
- Can control order of questions
- Greater control over participant – you know who has provided data
- Can produce supplementary data more readily.

Weaknesses of structured interviews
- Costly and time consuming
- Lack of anonymity
- Interviewer bias
- Participants have less control
- Involves the use of expensive equipment
- More intrusive
- Not always as acceptable to participants
- Possibility of participants giving dishonest answers or answering in a way designed to please the researcher.

Further reading

Murphy-Black, T. Questionnaires. In: DFS Cormack (ed.) *The Research Process in Nursing*, 4th edn. Blackwell Science: Oxford, 2000: pp. 301–13.

Oppenheim, AN. *Questionnaire Design, Interviewing and Attitude Measurement*, 2nd edn. Pinter Publishing: London, 1992.

Parahoo, K. Questionnaires: use, value and limitations. *Nurse Researcher* **1**(2): 4–15, 1993.

Quantitative data analysis

This type of data analysis uses statistical procedures to give meaning to information collected during the research.

Descriptive statistics

These are used to describe and merge data. The main descriptive statistics used are:
- Measures of central tendency – mean, median, and mode.
- Distribution – standard deviation and range.

Numerical data may also be described using graphs, tables, or figures. It is important to know about level of measurement before you describe your data.

Level of measurement

This is a system for categorizing different types of measures. There are four levels of measurement: nominal, ordinal, interval, and ratio. Although different measures may use different levels of measurement, it is possible to convert data to represent a different level of measurement, for example if you request people's ages by using categories 21–30 and so forth this is nominal data; if you ask people to state their age, this is interval data.

Inferential statistics

These allow researchers to draw conclusions from their data. Broadly speaking there are three types of quantitative research design – surveys, correlational, and experimental design. Within each of these designs the quantitative researcher usually tests relationships between variables.

What is a statistical test?

An analytical procedure that allows a researcher to determine the likelihood that results obtained from a sample reflect true population results, according to the laws of probability.

Why use a statistical test?
- To determine if you can generalize the results beyond the sample studied.
- To determine whether obtained results are statistically significant or not.
- To determine if you can reject the null hypothesis that states that the variables are not related.

Factors influencing the choice of statistical test
- Level of measurement.
- Sample size and sampling method.
- The degree of variance in responses to the dependent variable.
- The research design.
- Number of independent variables.
- Number of levels of the independent variables.

Patrick Callaghan, Professor of Mental Health Nursing, University of Nottingham & Nottinghamshire Healthcare NHS Trust

Level of significance (probability level)

This is the level at which the researcher is prepared to reject or accept the null hypothesis. The level of significance is the probability of the researcher's results occurring by chance. It also gives information on the potential of research results to be generalized beyond the sample studied. The significance level is usually expressed as follows.

$P < 0.05$ – the researcher will reject the null hypothesis if the results are significant 95 times out of a 100.

$P < 0.01$ – the researcher will reject the null hypothesis if the results are significant 99 times out of a 100.

$P < 0.10$ – the researcher will reject the null hypothesis if the results are significant 90 times out of a 100.

For example: A researcher compares Cognitive Behaviour Therapy (CBT) with Supportive Psychotherapy (SP) in treating the negative symptoms of Schizophrenia. Imagine the researcher analysed the results from this study and found that CBT was better than SP in reducing negative symptoms and the results were statistically significant at $p < 0.05$. This means that there is a 5 in 100 chance that negative symptoms were reduced by something other than CBT.

Key issues in quantitative data analysis

Selection of appropriate statistical test

Before running a statistical test on research data, you must check that your research design meets the requirements of the test you propose to use. There are two broad types of statistical tests: parametric and non-parametric. Within each of these types there are many different tests. Parametric tests are the strongest tests, and most researchers prefer to use these tests on their data where possible. However, the rules for running parametric tests are stricter than those for non-parametric tests.

Parametric versus non-parametric tests

The research community has debated at length how strict one should be in applying the rule regarding level of measurement for the use of parametric tests. You can apply both parametric and non-parametric tests to ordinal data. If the results are contradictory then you should report the results of the non-parametric test.

Requirements for using parametric tests

Your data should meet the following requirements before you may use a parametric test:

- Your level of measurement should be *interval* at least (with the above in mind).
- Your scores should be normally distributed.
- The variability in your data should be homogeneous.

When designing the study, you need to pay particular attention to the level of measurement of instruments that you use, and of demographic data that you collect. Normal distribution and variance can be tackled by sampling techniques that maximise representativeness of your sample.

Statistical Power Analysis

This is a procedure for reducing the likelihood of making a Type two error (see opposite). It determines the probability of obtaining a significant result. There are four components of a power analysis. The researcher must know at least three of these beforehand. These components are:

- Level of significance (see below)
- Population effect size
- Sample size
- Power

Researchers use power analysis to determine the sample size needed to demonstrate significant results and to determine the power of a statistical test. Achieving statistical power is not simply a matter of increasing sample size. It can also be achieved by: ensuring that treatment conditions of an independent variable are different from control conditions; selecting dependent variables that are realistically related to independent variables; and the timing of measuring a dependent variable.

Level of significance

This is the level at which you are prepared to reject or accept the null hypotheses. The level of significance is really the probability of your

Patrick Callaghan, Professor of Mental Health Nursing, University of Nottingham & Nottinghamshire Healthcare NHS Trust

results occurring by chance, or as a result of your research design. It will also provide information on the potential of your findings to be generalized beyond your sample. Obviously, the lower the level of significance the more likely you are to reject the null hypotheses. In most quantitative social and behavioural science research, the level of significance is normally set at 5% or $p < 0.05$.

Type 1 and Type 2 errors

A Type 1 error is when you say that two variables were related to one another when in fact they were not. This is most likely to occur when the researcher fails to pick up differences between the groups at the beginning of the research. A Type 2 error is made when the researcher concludes that the variables are not related, when in fact they are. When these errors occur, differences that appear between the groups at the end of the research are interpreted as arising from the research design. In fact, they were apparent from the outset of the research. Type 1 and Type 2 errors will mislead people and can have serious consequences e.g. in a randomized controlled trial testing the effect of a new drug.

Avoiding Type 1 and Type 2 errors

- Adequate sample size
- Representative sample
- Appropriate research design
- Homogeneous sample

Establishing the psychometric status of research measures

This may be the first stage of analysis after your descriptive statistics. It will involve calculating coefficients to determine the reliability and concurrent validity of your measure(s).

Types of analyses

There are two broad categories of quantitative data analyses:

- *Bivariate analyses* are tests that
  - look for differences between groups as defined by one variable, on scores on another variable.
  - test associations (relationships or correlations) between scores on two variables.
- *Multivariate analyses* are tests that
  - look for differences between two or more groups on a number of dependent variables.
  - test associations between scores on a number of variables.

Further reading

Hicks, CM. Research and Statistics: *A practical introduction for nurses*. Prentice Hall: London, 1990.

Kanji, GK. *100 statistical tests*. Sage: London, 1999.

Polit, DF, Beck, C. *Nursing Research, Principles and Methods*, 6th edn. Lippincott: Philadelphia PA, 2004.

Ethical issues in research

All human behaviour is conducted within ethical and moral codes, and the practice of research is not different in this respect. Researchers must ensure that they are adhering to universally acknowledged ethical principles – such as those described in the Helsinki Declaration of 1952 – in the conduct of their research. It is these principles that are described here.

The principle of beneficence

Research should yield benefits. Mental health nursing research should ultimately benefit people who use mental health services. People who participate in research must be protected from harm and exploitation. An assessment of the risk/benefit ratio should help researchers and those who govern the conduct of research to ensure that the principle of beneficence is upheld.

Principle of respect for human dignity

Researchers must respect the rights of participants and ensure that their dignity is upheld at all times during the research process. Participants have the right to self-determination and should be fully informed of what researchers require of them, and why.

The principle of justice

People who participate in research have the right to fair treatment and privacy.

Informed consent

Researchers must not enrol people in research who have not given informed consent to participate. To be fully informed, potential participates must know – their status, the purpose of the study, the type of data that will be collected, the nature of the commitment expected of them, how they were selected for participation, what exactly they must do, and what are the potential benefits and risks of participating. Participants should know that their consent is voluntary and that they can withdraw from the research at any time with impunity, and that alternatives to treatment that might have been given for research purposes will be available to them if they withdraw from the research. Participants should also be given information on who to contact to discuss the research and their participation. They should be informed that information they provide to researchers is confidential, unless this information threatens the health and safety of others.

Working with vulnerable people

There are additional safeguards when research includes participants who are classed as vulnerable. Vulnerable groups include children, people living with learning or physical disabilities, mental illness, terminal illness, pregnant women, and those who are institutionalized.

Patrick Callaghan, Professor of Mental Health Nursing, University of Nottingham & Nottinghamshire Healthcare NHS Trust

External review and approval
Researchers must comply with the ethical procedures of their respective governments. Research with humans and animals should not be conducted until a Research Ethics Committee approves it. The Department of Health in England requires that researchers adhere to its research governance framework which can be found on its website at www.dh.gov.uk.

Writing research proposals

General points
- Write in the future tense
- Tailor proposal to guidelines
- Structure will be similar to research report
- Be succinct and focused
- A proposal may change after consultation with supervisor or advisers.

Stages involved in writing a research proposal
- Abstract – a synopsis of the whole proposal
- Significance of the proposed research
- Background or literature review
- Aims and objectives
- Research questions or hypotheses (if appropriate)
- Methods
- Design
- Sample and sampling
- Data collection
- Procedure
- Data analysis
- Dissemination
- Ethical issues.

Establishing significance of the proposed study
- Relate to deficits in existing literature
- Relate to policy issues/recommendations: local, national, international
- Highlight innovations e.g. of topic or methods
- Target to interests of the funding body
- Show clearly how proposed research will improve practice, education, management, research
- Contribution to theory
- General applicability.

Background
- Review important existing literature – be selective
- Show how proposed research builds upon or extends existing work
- Mount a coherent, convincing argument for the proposed research that is obvious to the reader.

Aims and objectives
- Be specific
- Be focused
- Objectives must be achievable
- Provide clear criteria against which proposed methods can be assessed.

Patrick Callaghan, Professor of Mental Health Nursing, University of Nottingham & Nottinghamshire Healthcare NHS Trust

Research aims, objectives, questions, or hypotheses should be
- Clear
- Succinct
- Achievable
- Specific
- Focused
- Related to methods.

Design
- Describe design
- Justify
- Adhere to criteria for well-designed studies e.g. CONSORT statement
- Sample and sampling
- Describe sample characteristics and size
- How it is to be accessed
- Determination of sample size
- Describe sampling method
- Ensure sample is representative – use probability sampling if possible
- Consider sampling issues for specific research approaches e.g. focus groups, action research
- Data collection
- Describe and justify data collection methods
- Address issues of reliability, validity, and credibility
- Ensure methods can be independently verifiable.

Procedure
- Describe in detail how attrition is dealt with e.g. setting, protocols
- Include pilot study.

Data analysis
- Describe in detail proposed analysis
- Describe exactly what analysis will yield
- Ensure systematic analysis
- Address issues of reducing bias
- How to resolve differences in interpretation if more than one person is analysing the data.

Dissemination
- Describe in detail
- Differentiate diffusion from dissemination
- State how to implement findings.

Identify ethical issues raised by proposed research
- State how ethical probity will be ensured
- Ethical approval almost always required
- Adhere to RGF.

Writing for publication

Many mental health nurses publish work in a variety of outlets such as journals, books, and web outlets. The publication may be a research report, a clinical case study, or an opinion piece. Getting published is a competitive and demanding process. The following may increase your chances of getting your work published.

Developing writing skills
- The art of writing is simplicity and clarity.
- Read examples of excellent writing – not just academic.
- Practice with short pieces.
- Use critical readers – seek feedback.
- Use manuals e.g. *The Writer's Manual*[3].
- Use software packages.
- Start at a basic level and then progress to more complex pieces.

Clarifying the focus of the paper
- Plan the paper.
- Have a succinct introduction.
- Remind yourself of the aim of the paper.
- Stick to the aim.
- Use section headings.
- Conclude succinctly.

Writing a research paper
Introduction and literature review
- Evaluate previous work.
- Identify knowledge gaps in previous work.
- Describe how your work addresses gaps in previous work.

Methods
- Structure into sections – follow the format or design of the particular publication.
- Sample – describe sample and sampling methods.
- Measures/data collection methods – state what were your data collections methods.
- Procedure – describe how the research was carried out exactly.
- Data analysis – describe how the data were analysed.
- Results – report the results.

Communicating research results
Follow sequence of aims, objectives, hypotheses if appropriate.
- Use illustrations.
- Avoid jargon – state exactly what results mean in lay terms.
- Give examples – direct quotes.
- Summarize results if they are lengthy.
- Use correct grammar.

Patrick Callaghan, Professor of Mental Health Nursing, University of Nottingham & Nottinghamshire Healthcare NHS Trust

General tips on using English correctly

- Don't use double negatives.
- Make each pronoun agree with its antecedent.
- Don't dangle participles.
- Don't use unnecessary commas.
- Verbs have to agree with their subject.
- Do not use sentence fragments.
- Try not to split infinitives.
- Use apostrophes correctly.
- Always read what you have written to see if you have left any words out.
- Correct spelling is essential.

Reference

3 Cook, R. *The Writer's Manual: A Step-by-Step Guide for Nurses and Other Health Profession-als*. Radcliffe Medical Press: Oxford, 1999.

Further reading

Lester, JD. *Writing Research Papers – A Complete Guide*, 8th edn. Harper Collins: New york, 1996.
Turabian, KL. *A Manual for Writers of Term Papers, Theses and Dissertations*, 6th edn. University of Chicago Press: Chicago IL, 1996.

Using research to improve practice

Mental health nursing is about promoting mental health, and caring for people using mental health services. The aim is to help people recover their ability to live relatively free from ill health. Mental health nursing research is about providing an evidence base to support the activities of mental health nurses, and others doing similar work. There is an overwhelming source of evidence-based information that nurses can use in their work. However there are key skills required in using this evidence to improve practice, not least of which is the ability to evaluate published research.

The term evaluate means to judge the worth or value of something. Evaluation requires a balanced critique during which you will identify strengths and weaknesses of published evidence. The CASP (Critical Appraisal Skills Programme) website[4] has checklists for evaluating different types of research reports. It is an indispensable source of useful information for evaluating published research.

General tips on evaluating published research
- Be as objective as possible.
- Do not insult the author(s) or question their competence.
- Be reasonable in your critique.
- Give specific examples of the strengths and limitations of the paper.
- Be sensitive in making negative statements – put yourself in the author's shoes.
- Try to justify your criticisms.
- Suggest alternatives.

Getting research into practice
What works?
- Academic detailing – lectures.
- Opinion leaders – Influential and credible people.
- Audit/feedback.
- Reminder systems.
- Patient mediated interventions.

Consistently effective interventions
- Educational outreach visits.
- Reminders.
- Multifacetted interventions (e.g. two or more of audit and feedback, reminders, local consensus processes, marketing).
- Interactive educational meetings.

Interventions of variables effectiveness
- Audit and feedback.
- Local opinion leaders.
- Local consensus processes.
- Patient mediated interventions.

Patrick Callaghan, Professor of Mental Health Nursing, University of Nottingham & Nottinghamshire Healthcare NHS Trust

Interventions that have little or no effect
- Educational materials.
- Didactic educational meetings.

The experiences of putting evidence into practice
Factors related to likelihood of success
- Sufficient resources (i.e. time. money, and skills).
- Benefits to front-line staff from the proposed change.
- Enough of the right people are on board early enough.
- Interactive approach linking research clearly to practice.

Key lessons
- Expect to take several years.
- Successful implementation requires pragmatism and flexibility.
- Start small and build incrementally.
- Use what is already there.
- Target enthusiasts first.

Outcomes
- Better relationships.
- Improved knowledge, systems, and skills.
- Practice change.
- Improved patent care.

Reference

4 Critical Appraisal Skills Programme website: www.phru.nhs.uk/CASP

Further reading

Benton, DC, Cormack, DFS. *Reviewing and evaluating the literature*. 2000. Cormack, DFS (ed.). *The Research Process in Nursing*, 4th edn. Blackwell Science: Oxford, 2000.

Bero, LA, Grilli, R, Grimshaw, JM, et al. Closing the gap between research and practice: an overview of systematic reviews of interventions to promote the implementation of research findings. *British Medical Journal* **317**: 465–8, 1997.

Cormack, DFS (ed.). *The Research Process in Nursing*, 4th edn. Blackwell Science: Oxford, 2000.

Greenhalgh, T. *How to read a paper: the basis of evidence-based medicine*. BMJ: London, 2001.

Wye, L, McClenahan, J. *Getting better with evidence: experiences of putting evidence into practice*. King's Fund: London, 2000.

Liaison mental health services

Liaison mental health services

Liaison mental health services (LMHS) provide support to non-mental health practitioners and services. They aim to meet the psychological and mental health needs of patients receiving primary treatment for a non-mental health problem. They may also offer services in emergency departments to patients whose presenting problem is one of mental distress. It is estimated that up to 65% of medical inpatients have psychiatric symptoms.

Evolution of liaison mental health services

Liaison mental health nursing was first developed in the USA. Liaison nurses were clinical specialists, offering support and education for general hospital nurses. They also provided care direct to patients and families.

Liaison mental health nursing in the United Kingdom developed in the 1990s. The first published evidence is of nurses in oncology units, followed by out-of-hours mental health provision in emergency departments.

The government's concern to reduce suicide rates provided impetus for the development of services in emergency departments and specific self-harm provision. Recent emphasis on twenty-four hour access to support for anyone with a mental health problem further increased the emergency department provision.

Structure of services

There are numerous models of LMHS: liaison nurses may work on their own or within a single disciplinary nurse led service. Alternatively, liaison nurses may work as part of a team, including some or all of these professionals:
- Psychiatrists
- Social workers
- Psychologists

There is little evidence supporting one model of LMHS over another.

Service provision varies from 9a.m.–5p.m. Monday to Friday to twenty-four hour services that are provided 365 days of the year.

Liaison nurses work across all age ranges, although other services are often age specific. Adult services are much more common than older adult or child and adolescent services.

📖 Working with children and adolescents

Evaluation of services

The majority of published information about liaison mental health services is descriptive. However, there is evidence that LMHS based in emergency departments ease the burden of general emergency department staff, help clients access mental health services, and reduce the re-admission rates of people with mental health problems. There is also evidence that general hospital nurses value the responsiveness and the ease of access of liaison nursing services.

Sarah Eales, City University, London

Further reading

Callaghan, P, Eales, S, Coats, TJ, et al. A review of the structure, process and outcome of liaison mental health services. *Journal of Psychiatric and Mental Health Nursing* **10**(2): 155-65, 2003.

The process of liaison mental health care

Liaison mental health nursing (LMHN) can take many forms. The most common is accepting a referral from another discipline, where there is a concern that the patient is showing signs of mental distress. This might be a known mental health problem, a psychological reaction to trauma, or a person with a suspected mental health problem presenting to the emergency department.

A model for service provision

Liaison mental health nurses usually offer a range of services, not just the assessment and treatment of individual patients.

Caplan[1] identified the following models of liaison mental health service provision:

Client-centered service – the direct assessment and treatment of a referred patient. Education is a secondary concern.

Programme-centered administrative service – this includes involvement in planning service delivery; for example, advice on drawing up policies to assist nurses with one to one observation in a general hospital setting.

Consultee-centered service – this involves working with the staff. Education is the primary concern here, rather than the individual patient. Nurses may lack the knowledge, skills, or confidence to work with a patient who has a mental health issue.

Consultee-centered administrative service – this involves ongoing support to maintain the mental health aspects of service delivery, for example follow-up visits to a ward or unit to review the implementation of training.

Client centered and consultee centered care are the most frequently provided services.

📖 Person-centered mental health nursing

The process of liaison mental health care

When a patient is referred to the nurse, (s)he should establish the reason for referral, the presenting complaint, any evidence of risk behaviour, and the expected outcome from the perspective of the referrer. The patient's consent for the referral should be obtained, except in emergency situations.

Once the referral is accepted, the nurse should:

• *Gather information* – obtain background information, including information from the GP and where relevant, the patient's mental health team. Friends and relatives may have important information on the development of the problem, and the patient's mental health history.

• *Assess* – undertake a thorough psychosocial assessment. It is important to consider the patient's perception of the problem, and its cause. A mental state examination and a thorough risk assessment should be given a high priority in the assessment process (📖 Mental health assessment).

Sarah Eales, City University, London

- *Formulate* – formulate a summary of the problems, including the identification of current and potential risk, including triggers that lead to an increase in risk (📖 Risk management).
- *Treatment* – identify a treatment plan, taking time to discuss the options with the referrer and the patient before making a decision. Treatment may include referral to other mental health or substance misuse services. Short-term supportive counselling and brief cognitive behavioural therapy may be provided by the liaison nurse (📖 Cognitive behaviour therapy, 📖 Motivational interviewing).
- *Follow-up* – on-going monitoring and treatment may be required. Repeating the mental state examination will help to determine the effectiveness of treatment and the reduction in symptoms.
- *Communication* – having identified if a problem is present, the nature of any risk and the treatment plan, it is important to ensure that the patient, the referrer and any other relevant professionals are aware of the outcome of the assessment (📖 Interpersonal communication).

Reference

1 Caplan, G. The Theory and Practice of Mental Health Consulation. London: Tavistock Publications 1970.

Liaison mental health nursing competencies

Liaison mental health nurses may hold responsibility for decisions to admit or discharge. They are likely to be senior clinical nurses banded at level seven. Working in the general hospital setting, they can be called to see patients whose primary problem lies outside their specialist area. Good relationships within different specialisms are paramount to ensure an understanding of the patient's primary problem.

There are a number of competencies of liaison mental health nursing, including effective documentation, that are common to mental health nurses in other areas, others are specific to LMHN.

Competencies

Liaison nurses need to be competent to undertake work in the following areas:
- Admission and discharge of patients.
- Assessment and management of risk and self-harm.
- Providing nursing advice on medication.
- Patients with complex or challenging presentations.
- Advice on legal and ethical issues, including capacity to consent (📖 Assessing capacity to consent).
- Treatment appropriate to the general hospital setting, including managing dual medical-psychological presentations and psychiatric emergencies.
- People with specific physical disorders, including knowledge of the psychological morbidity associated with specific physical disorders.
- Working with specific physical and psychosomatic disorders (📖 People with specific psychosomatic disorders).
- Mothers and babies – perinatal care, including postnatal depression.
- Substance misuse – including identification of symptoms of withdrawal (📖 Working with the person with substance misuse).
- Accurate records, documentation, and report writing, including preparing discharge summaries (📖 Record keeping).
- Evaluation of liaison mental health nursing interventions.

Sarah Eales, City University, London

Further reading

Hart, C, Eales, S (eds.). *A Competence Framework for Liaison Mental Health Nursing*. London Liaison Mental Health Nurses Special Interest Group, 2004. [Unpublished]

Working with specific physical and psychosomatic disorders

Nurses in a general hospital may require assistance in managing the psychological consequences of physical health problems. Nurses may be fearful of mental health issues; they may feel that they lack the knowledge and skills to meet psychological needs, or that they simply do not have the time. Some patients present with physical symptoms, where no underlying physical cause can be identified; frequently, these patients are suffering from a psychosomatic disorder. Liaison nurses have a role in the education of the nursing staff, assessment, planning, and treatment of co-morbidity and psychosomatic illness.

Epidemiology

Illnesses such as HIV and end-stage renal failure have high incidences of accompanying psychological distress. Over 10% of medical admissions are for deliberate self-harm. Depression is evident in between 25% and 45% of general hospital patients. Approximately 1 in 10 patients admitted for an acute condition will have an acute confusional state accompanying their medical condition. Up to 50% of symptoms in an outpatient department may be unexplained by physical causes.

Adjustment reactions and depression

It is quite usual to feel some psychological distress when in hospital. A change of environment, the absence of friends and relatives, and a concern about treatment and prognosis, can all lead to stress, anxiety, and fear.

The liaison nurse needs to educate and assist the general hospital team in determining what is normal and what an abnormal reaction is. Prolonged problems adjusting to physical illness may lead to depression, the most common mental illness. The liaison nurse has a key role in assessing, identifying, and recommending treatment for depression. They cannot rely on normal indicators such as sleep disturbance and loss of appetite, as these may be present as a consequence of the physical health problem. Untreated depression may delay recovery, interfere with activity such as physiotherapy, and prolong the physical illness. Symptoms such as withdrawal, pessimism, and guilt may be better indicators of depression in patients with physical health problems. The Hospital Anxiety and Depression Scale is a validated tool for use in assessment.

Acute confusional states (delirium)

Symptoms of acute confusion include:
- Disorientation to time and place.
- Psychotic symptoms, such as paranoia and hallucinations.
- Challenging behaviour.

Sarah Eales, City University, London

Acute confusion often has an underlying physical cause, for example:
• Infections, such as chest infections and urinary tract infections.
• Constipation.
• Hypoxia.

The presentation may appear to indicate a psychiatric disorder, but the onset is usually very rapid, rather than incremental. Liaison nurses need to be able to identify acute confusion and help nurses manage the symptoms, whilst the underlying physical cause is treated.

Assessing capacity to consent

Every patient has the legal and ethical right to decide whether to enter into a particular type of care or treatment. The only exception is under specific sections of the Mental Health Act (1983).

Consent may be written, verbal, or non-verbal depending on the circumstances. The person carrying out a procedure must gain consent and remains responsible for this. There are very few exceptions to this requirement to obtain a patient's consent. The Department of Health and each local health trust will have specific guidance on gaining consent. The liaison nurse may be asked to assist in the assessment of capacity and/or in the gaining of consent.

Principles of consent

The patient must:
• Have the capacity to make the decision.
• Be provided with enough information to make the decision.
• Not be acting under duress.

An attempt should be made to obtain consent from every patient for all interventions. If the patient is unable to consent, treatment may still be given in the patients 'best interests'.

No-one can consent on behalf of an adult patient, although when a patient lacks capacity their friends and relatives may be able to assist the professional in making a 'best interest' decision. Advanced directives made by a patient when capable, should be reasonably honoured. Disagreement within the multidisciplinary team about 'best interests' treatment and care will often lead to a request for a legal review of the issue.

Assessment of capacity to consent

To assess capacity, the liaison nurse needs to be sure that the patient:
• Can comprehend and retain the information needed to make a decision
• Is able to use and weigh the information in the decision making process.[2]

The NICE guidelines on self-harm break this assessment down further. To demonstrate capacity to give or withhold consent, the individual should be able to:
• Understand in simple language what the treatment is, its purpose and nature, and why it is being proposed.
• Understand its principal benefits, risks, and alternatives.
• Understand in broad terms what will be the consequences of not receiving the proposed treatment.
• Retain the information for long enough to make an effective decision.
• Believe the information.
• Weigh the information in the balance.
• Make a free choice.

Sarah Eales, City University, London

Patients frequently refuse to consent because they do not understand the proposed treatment, and would benefit from further information. Refusal of treatment does not indicate a lack of capacity. Capacity may fluctuate in a patient, and for each procedure, lack of capacity should not be assumed.

Detailed documentation of any assessment and the decisions made is extremely important. The local health trust will have forms that need to be completed.

Reference

2 Department of Health. Good Practice in consent Implementation Guide: consent to examination or treatment. DoH: London, 2001. See also: www.dh.gov.uk/consent

Further reading

The British Psychological Society and The Royal College of Psychiatrists. Self-harm. *The short-term physical and psychological management and secondary prevention of self-harm in primary and secondary care. Guideline* 16. NICE: London, 2004.

National Occupational Standards for Mental Health

Practising in a reflective and professionally appropriate manner

The concept of reflection has been around for several years. It is considered an accessible form of learning for nurses regardless of what point they are at in their career. There are a number of different models to choose from to aid reflection (see below). Each model has a number of common areas which inform the nursing process; these can provide evidence of continuing professional education and learning in accordance with PREP requirements (UKCC, 1999). There are many definitions in the literature of reflection, most however agree that it is an active, conscious process.

📖 Clinical Supervision

Reflection is often initiated when the individual practitioner encounters some problematic aspect of practice and attempts to make sense of it.
   Reflection can also help achieve the following:
• It helps to bridge the gap between theory and practice.
• It shows the interrelation of skills and knowledge – it is an expansion of cognitive learning.
• Knowledge obtained from reflection can shift the emphasis of care to the human side of nursing.
• It encourages practitioners to critically evaluate their behaviour, beliefs, and ideas on practice.

Undertaking some form of reflection will benefit a nurse's practice. It will ensure that their intuition or the common practice they follow is constantly in keeping with current theory and acceptable practice.

Models of reflection

There are a number of different models including the following:

Callister argues that when we reflect on clinical events we expand our cognitive learning. In undertaking this process the biomedical model becomes less important and the emphasis shifts to the human side of nursing.[1]

Ramsden feels that through reflection we can understand people's motivation, and their perceptions as these are intrinsically linked to their individual experiences.[2]

Jasper states that reflection can help bridge the theory-practice gap.[3]

Benner sees reflection as essential to nurses throughout their career, although she also holds the opinion that a practitioner cannot always explain their expert knowledge to others as it has become internalized.[4]

Rolfe stresses the importance of being able to distinguish between practical knowledge (knowing how) and theoretical knowledge (knowing why). He argues that nurses should use reflection to build new theories that can be tested and re-tested in practice.[5]

Betsey Scott, East London and the City Mental Health NHS Trust

Role of the mental health nurse

- Develop your knowledge and practice.
- Promote effective communication for and about individuals.
- Relate to and interact with individuals.
- Support individuals with specific communication needs.
- Support individuals to communicate using interpreting and translation services.
- Relate to families, parents, and carers.
- Promote the values and principles underpinning best practice.
- Maintain and manage records and reports.
- Support colleagues to relate to individuals.
- Promote the values and principles underpinning best practice.
- Promote effective communication and relationships with people who are troubled or distressed.

The full version of the Mental Health National Occupational Standards is available at www.skillsforhealth.org.uk

References

1 Callister, LC. The use of student journals in nursing education: making meaning out of clinical experience. *Journal of Nursing Education* **32**(4): 185–86, 1993.

2 Ramsden, P. Learning to teach in Higher Education Rontledge: London 1994.

3 Jasper, M. Beginning reflective practice. Cheltenham, Nelson Thomas, 1998.

4 Benner. From Notice to Expert. Prentice Hall, USA: 1984.

5 Rolfe, G. Expanding nursing knowledge, understanding and reflecting on your prentice. Oxford: Buterworth–Heinemann, 1998.

Further reading

Bulman, C, Reflective Practice in Nursing: the growth of the professional practitioner. Blackwell: Oxford, 2004.

Freshwater, D. Transforming Nursing through Reflective Practice. Blackwell: Oxford, 2005.

Jasper, M, Thorpes, N. Foundations in Nursing and Health Care; beginning reflective practice. Nelson Thornes: Cheltenham, 2003.

Enabling access to mental health services

A key concept in mental health care is the promotion of independence and autonomy. This includes enabling those with mental health needs to access services and facilities to aid their recovery or to maintain their mental health as is stipulated in the NSF through 24-hour access to mental health services.

The list of services and resources given below is not exhaustive but available throughout England and Wales at a local level as is the minimum required for service users.

The health team

The team involved in a person's care at a time of crisis should be up to date and knowledgeable about the resources and services available to support people in crisis, during recovery and beyond.

The Internet

There are many websites giving information on services and facilities, including the Department of Health's website, websites for mental health trusts in England, and primary and secondary care trusts. There is a dedicated website for mental health nurses and students, providing information, resources, news, and jobs.[6]

GP and other primary care providers

GPs are often the first port of call for people with mental health needs; they should be able to give information and advice on services, and refer onwards where necessary. Some larger practices have a mental health professional based in the surgery.

Strategic Health Authorities (SHA)

SHAs are responsible for all Trusts and NHS services within a geographical area; they are able to give information on all health care services in this area for people with mental health needs and other needs such as dentistry and family planning clinics.

PALS

Every NHS Trust will have a Patient Advice and Liaison Service (PALS) officer who can give advice and information. You do not have to be a service user of a particular trust to access information from a PALS service.

NHS Direct

Health queries can be answered by telephone (0845 4647) or by logging onto the NHS direct online website (www.nhsdirect.nhs.uk). For users whose first language is not English, a confidential interpreting service can be accessed by phoning the telephone number above and stating the language of choice at the start of the call.

Johanna Turner, Performance Panel Coordinator and Legal Advisor, Newham PCT, London

Charities and other independent organizations

These include voluntary organizations and self help and support groups providing information, support and independent advice e.g. Mind, Sane, and the Alzheimer's disease Society. Local branches of some of the National organisations such as MIND often have local directories of services specifically for mental health service users, and their carers. This is an invaluable resource for mental health professionals.

Role of the mental health nurse

- Support individuals to represent their own needs and wishes at decision making forums.
- Provide advice and information to those who enquire about mental health needs and related services.
- Work with service providers to support people with mental health needs in ways which promote their rights.
- Assist individuals to evaluate and contact support networks.
- Enable support networks to develop their effectiveness.

The full version of the Mental Health National Occupational Standards is available at www.skillsforhealth.org.uk

Reference

6 www.mentalhealthnurse.co.uk

Providing mental health services which support families and carers

Under the Carers' (Recognition and Services) Act 1995, carers have a right to an assessment of their own needs. The Mental Health Bill also recognizes that carers play a crucial role.

Assessments of carers' needs are the responsibility of local social services departments although they can be completed by any qualified member of a community mental health team. In addition, the National Service Framework for Mental Health, standard six, states that all individuals who provide regular and substantial care for a person on the care programme approach (CPA) should:
- Have an assessment of their caring, physical, and mental health needs, repeated on at least an annual basis.
- Have their own written care plan, which is given to them and implemented in discussion with them.

Support can be accessed in a variety of ways by carers and their families including:
- Advice and information from secondary care services e.g. a primary nurse/named nurse should be able to provide advice about what support is available for carers while the clients with mental health problems who are in crisiane in hospital.
- Organizations such as Mind offer fact sheets, links to other organizations and voluntary groups, who can offer support and guidance including financial and legal assistance, respite, and emotional support.
- Websites which might be helpful include:
  - Mind – www.mind.org.uk
  - Rethink (previously known as the National Schizophrenic Fellowship) – www.rethink.org
  - Government websites – www.carers.gov.uk
- In a crisis, carers may contact the Samaritans – a confidential, 24-hour service providing emotional support for those people experiencing distress and despair (Telephone: 08457 909090).
- Social Services carry out assessments of carers' needs (see above). Find the contact details of your local authority's social service department either from the local telephone directory, the library, or from your GP or hospital staff. The assessment focuses on how people can be supported to continue caring, if they wish to.

Role of the mental health nurse
- Help parents and carers to acquire and use skills to protect and take care of children and young people.
- Support families in their own home.
- Work in collaboration with carers in the caring role.
- Assess the needs of carers and families of individuals with mental health needs.

Johanna Turner, Performance Panel Coordinator and Legal Advisor, Newham PCT, London

- Develop, implement, and review programmes of support for carers and families.
- Establish, sustain, and disengage from relationships with the families of children and young people.
- Empower families, carers, and others to support individuals with mental health needs.
- Establish, sustain, and disengage from relationships with the families of older people with mental health needs.
- Support families in maintaining relationships in their wider social structures and environment.
- Work with families, carers, and individuals during times of crisis.

These expectations are in keeping with the principles and codes of professional practice and must adhere to the principles of confidentiality. The full version of the Mental Health National Occupational Standards is available at www.skillsforhealth.org.uk

Further reading

Lefley, HP. *Family Care Giving in Mental Illness*. Sage Publications:, 1996 (USA).
Okun, F. Understanding Diverse families: what practitioners need to know. Guilford Press: 1998. New York.

Assessing individual needs for programmes of care

Assessments may take place in primary, secondary, or tertiary care. A comprehensive assessment should ensure that strategies, services, and planned care delivery will assist in a swift recovery from crisis or possibly prevent a crisis occurring. Assessment is a fundamental skill for all mental health nurses.

The holistic needs of the individual include a person's physical, psychological, social, cultural, and spiritual well-being.

The assessment process

A thorough assessment process will involve the following factors:
- Reason for referral (who, why, current concerns, any previous concerns).
- Individuals perception (why they think they have been referred/are being assessed; purpose of the assessment).
- Individuals views on current mental health and social situation (recent changes, occupation, relationships/friendships, lifestyle).
- Physical health (general health, illnesses, previous history, appetite, weight, alcohol, tobacco, street drugs; list any prescribed medication with comments on effectiveness).
- Obtaining the views of the family, carers, and friends. This should be done with the expressed consent of the person being assessed (it may be necessary to consult the parents or legal guardians of children or young people).
- The needs of any carers as detailed in the National Service Framework for Mental Health.
- A comprehensive risk assessment; this is one of the key skills for mental health professionals (suicidal ideation/acts, self harm, threats of violence to others/property). 📖 Risk Assessment.
- Spiritual health (religion, culture, ethnicity).
- Mental state (hallucinations, delusions, sleep pattern, concentration, thought processes, cognition). 📖 Experience of mental illness.

Where possible all aspects of the assessment should be corroborated through another source such as the GP, referral source, or other professional.

Formulation

At the end of the assessment the nurse needs to draw all the information together to include a nursing diagnosis where possible in the form of a summary:
- Develop an action plan with the client as to what the next steps could be, giving choices and options as appropriate.
- Ensure that individuals are referred to the specific services that they need, both those identified by the assessor and by the person being assessed.

Vince Turner, North East London Mental Health Trust

Role of the mental health nurse

- Identify the physical health needs of individuals with mental health needs.
- Assess the need for intervention and present assessments of individuals' needs and related risks.
- Refer individuals to mental health and/or other services.
- Assess individuals mental health and related needs.
- Assess individuals' needs and circumstances and evaluate the risk of abuse, failure to protect and harm to self and others.

The full version of the Mental Health National Occupational Standards is available at www.skillsforhealth.org.uk

The risk assessment process

A risk assessment should pull together three main strands – the risk posed to self, to others, and from others. The emphasis of risk assessment should be on a client-centered perspective, and it is important to view it as an ongoing systematic process that is contributed to by the multi-disciplinary team as with the service user and carers.

At a minimum a risk assessment must incorporate:

- Usual behaviour patterns.
- Past history of risk behaviour (to self, property, others).
- Demographic factors (age, gender, socioeconomic status).
- Substance abuse.
- Acute psychiatric symptoms e.g. command hallucination, mania.

Within the process of risk assessment it is necessary to plan ahead for intervention to manage identified risks. Any intervention must strive to produce a therapeutic outcome, using the least restrictive means, leading to a recovery from crisis. Risk is a fluid process, informed by the changing needs of the person with mental health problems and is consequently under constant review.

Further reading

Sainsbury's Centre for Mental Health. Pulling together: the future roles and training of mental health staff. SCMH: London, 1997.

Tunmore, R. Practitioner assessment skills. In: T Thompson, P Mathias (eds.) *Lyttles Mental Health and Disorder*, 3rd edn.: 2000: p. 488.

Planning and reviewing care programmes for people with mental health needs

It is important to work with individuals and families to ensure that the care planned relates to their own perceived care needs, as well as to the professional's identification of their needs. People are more likely to engage with services if they feel they have ownership of the process and if they have contributed significantly to their own recovery. It is difficult to engage somebody who has not had the opportunity to take any responsibility for his or her own health needs.

The care programme needs to be written in a language which the individual, their carers, and family finds easy to understand. It should be clear, unambiguous, and specific in terms of what interventions are to be delivered by whom, when, where, and how the care will be evaluated.

Planned care needs to reflect the holistic approach used in the assessment considering all aspects of an individual, such as the physical, spiritual, social, cultural, and psychological.

The professional may have statutory and legal duties within the care programme; these should be balanced with the needs and preferences of the individual.

Benefits of a care programme

Some of the benefits of having a care plan include:
- Assists in setting and achieving goals.
- Encourages the client to be involved in their care.
- Manages long term care in a clear, concise way.
- Provides an essential checklist to ensure continuity of care.
- Prompts the client to take more responsibility for their care needs.
- Encourages a team approach to the client-centred plan.
- Focuses on improving and maintaining health rather than waiting for illness onset.
- Increases client and carer awareness of which services are needed and why.
- May provide life-saving information in crisis.

Crisis plan

A crisis plan needs to be discussed and developed with the service user. This should include information on people to contact, and on what support and practical help will be available for carers and families at the point of crisis. Where necessary the statutory duties of professionals need to be made explicit e.g. when assessment under the Mental Health Act (1983) may be necessary. Any crisis plan should incorporate an evaluation method for assessing the effectiveness of the plan after the event, and making changes as necessary.

Vince Turner, North East London Mental Health Trust

Role of the mental health nurse

- Contribute to care planning and review.
- Contribute to assessing the needs of individuals for therapeutic programmes to enable them to manage their behaviour.
- Access individual needs and preferences.
- Develop, implement, and review care plans with individuals.
- Coordinate, monitor, and review service responses to meet individuals' needs and circumstances.
- Work with individuals with mental health needs to negotiate and agree plans for addressing those needs.
- Respond to crisis situations.
- Maintain active continuing contact with individuals and work with them to monitor their mental health needs.

The full version of the Mental Health National Occupational Standards is available at www.skillsforhealth.org.uk

Review

Planning and reviewing care should be a fluid ongoing process. Professionals should be responsive to changes in a person's health; changes and amendments should be in consultation with the individual, and where necessary the multi-disciplinary team. The minimum requirement for enhanced level care programme review is annually.

Further reading

Bernan Associates. *Factors Influencing the Implementation of the Care Programme Approach.* HMSO: London, 1993.

Following through on care programmes for people with mental health needs

People must feel engaged in their care programme if they are to take ownership of it and actively participate in their care planning and review. Care delivery should focus on evidence-based practice, which is clinically effective. Clinical effectiveness is described as the extent to which specific clinical interventions, when deployed in the field for a particular patient or population, do what they are intended to do, that is maintain and improve health and secure the greatest possible health gain from available resources.

Role of the mental health nurse

All mental health staff are in the position of planning care via the CPA regardless of where the service user is within the service – i.e. at home, in an acute setting, in residential care, and must be skilled in some or all of the following areas:

- **Medicines management:** is complex and will not be the role of all care staff, only those designated to undertake this activity, and applies to all medication used for and by individuals, both prescribed and non-prescribed.
- **Planning and reviewing the effectiveness of therapeutic interventions with individuals with mental health needs:** Therapeutic interventions should reflect a holistic approach to care, and respond to an individual's needs. Qualified therapists providing therapy as a component of the CPA integrate their work with other practitioners' promoting the holistic nature of health and social well-being.
- **Reinforce positive behavioural goals during relationships with individuals:** Everyone responds to positive comments, and it is important that service users are given constructive feedback on their progress. Achievements must be recognized, and an overly critical approach avoided.
- **Contribute to the assessment of needs and the planning, evaluation, and review of individualized programmes of care for individuals:** Working as a member of an inter-disciplinary team to achieve agreed objectives with service users; contribute to the assessment planning and evaluation of individualised programmes of care, as agreed on a case-by-case basis.
- **Implement specific parts of individualized programmes of care:** As the care coordinator/named nurse/primary nurse you will be one of the main points of contact with service users undertaking specific individualised programmes of care. Where there is a conflict of interest it is important to ensure that the service users' rights are promoted involving advocacy services where necessary. Where appropriate, individuals, their family, or carers, should be given information on and/or training in the relevant skills, so that they can continue to use the therapies that were helpful, after the crisis has passed.

Vince Turner, North East London Mental Health Trust

• **Promote the benefits of activities to improve physical health and well-being and support the individual in access to services:** The physical health care of service users is often neglected and needs to form a central part of any care programme to include routine screening e.g. weight, blood pressure; health promotion e.g. diet, exercise; and routine health care e.g. dental treatment, chiropody for those with diabetes.

The full version on the Mental Health National Occupational Standards is available at www.skillsforhealth.org.uk

Further reading

Heaton, J. *Building Basic Therapeutic Skills: a practice guide*. John Wiley & Son: 1998. Chichester, UK.

Supporting people with mental health needs in managing their lives

It is estimated that at any one time, one in six adults suffers from some form of mental illness.[7] For most people, the experience of mental illness is distressing; it may have negative and far-reaching effects on every aspect of life, e.g. family problems, employment and social life, poverty, and discrimination issues.

Mental health professionals must be able to understand these problems and experiences, and their effects on the lives of service users. Repper and Perkins suggest much would be gained if mental health services utilized a 'social disability model' outlook on mental illness, with a focus on helping people to adapt and live with their illness.[8]

Mental illness and recovery from mental illness is complex and very individual; it is suggested that recovery not only involves overcoming the effects of the illness, but also the effect of the social exclusion that occurs. The government's Social Exclusion Unit has published several fact sheets giving practical solutions to promote social inclusion.

The role of the mental health nurse

- A sustained and consistent relationship with staff is beneficial to service users. A large survey carried out by Rethink found that people said being able to talk about their problems, caring, positive and reassuring staff, and being treated with respect, were the factors that helped them most during their experience of mental illness.[9]
- Mental health workers must take a person's wider circumstances into consideration if they are to support them. Housing, employment, finances, education, family role, social contacts, and spirituality are some of the issues to consider at each stage. Services must also be responsive to issues of gender, ethnicity, and sexuality.
- It is vital that staff consider each individual's personal development and aspirations, and focus on what is meaningful for them, listening to what they say about the way they want to live, and then offering options. Staff need to think creatively and beyond medication and admission, to ensure that the care plan reflects the service user's perspective and that of their social supports.
- Health and social services staff should work collaboratively, establishing links with other local services in order to access and make use of these services. This can ensure that individual needs are met and that people get the services that make a real difference to their lives, for example, disability living allowance and housing benefit. Service users must be supported in gaining access to wider opportunities within their communities, and not just rely on specific mental health provision.
- Person-centered planning is essential to supporting people to manage their lives. The focus is on promoting independence and helping people to build upon their personal assets and become empowered to take control of their lives.

The full version of the Mental Health National Occupational Standards is available at www.skillsforhealth.org.uk

Stephanie Tannis, East London and the City Mental Health NHS Trust

Supporting social inclusion

Mental health workers need to examine their own attitudes and beliefs toward service users, to work in partnership with and treat individuals with respect and dignity in order to help facilitate their social inclusion (Repper and Perkins 2003).

Mental health workers have an important role in assisting people to build, improve, and maintain their social relationships. The development of a trusting relationship with service users based on recovery and empowerment is at the core of mental health nursing. Nurses are well positioned to recognize the importance of hope and to inspire hope in people's lives. They are also well-positioned to challenge stigma and inequalities and to be an advocate for service users.

Statutory and voluntary sectors of the community must recognize that each has a responsibility to work towards the inclusion of vulnerable members. Effective collaboration across different sectors, and the recognition of the complex needs of service users is paramount to promoting the social inclusion of service users with multiple needs.

For example, mental health and substance misuse agencies (statutory or independent) work in partnership to support people with mental health problems and substance misuse issues. Social services and health services work jointly with specialist services to provide comprehensive care packages for people who have disabilities and mental health problems (Social Exclusion Unit Fact sheet 2, 2004).

References

7 Office of the Deputy Prime Minister. Mental Health and Social Exclusion: Social Exclusion Unit Report. ODPM: London, 2004.

8 Repper, J, Perkins, P. *Social Inclusion and Recovery*. Bailliere Tindall: Edinburgh, 2003.

9 Rethink website: www.rethink.org/research

Supporting people with mental health needs in managing social situations and interactions with others

The experience of mental illness may reduce an individual's ability to form and maintain social relationships. Social support is important for well-being and inclusion; and mental health staff have an important role in enabling service users to develop, improve, maintain, and benefit from these relationships.[10,11]

Mental health services must ensure that their services are inclusive and promote opportunities within the wider community. Partnership working enables links between community services and trans-referral arrangements whereby service users can benefit from wider experiences. The ODPM suggests there must be a recognition of the diversity of needs around gender, ethnicity, and culture.[12] Services should reflect this and if needed, arrange for specialist support from other sectors of the community.

The role of the mental health nurse

Mental health staff can support people by:

- Building and maintaining social networks, by acting as role models in their interactions with service users and other colleagues. Offering social skills training and using role play can be helpful, as service users have the opportunity to practice social interaction in a safe environment with people they trust. The support offered to manage social situations depends on the needs of the individual and the circumstances.
- Accessing opportunities that the person values by offering information, choice, and practical support e.g. contacting and attending with them. Asking service users what they want to do is important.
- Assisting service users to have a routine and to use a diary.
  A step-by-step plan of tackling stressful social situations can be useful e.g. gradual exposure to at least one social situation a week and building up over time, while simultaneously learning and exploring coping strategies.
- Providing skills training (e.g. assertiveness and confidence building), motivation and consistent support. They can also provide advocacy, befriending, and support to enable people to make opportunities for social contact.

The full version of the Mental Health National Occupational Standards is available at www.skillsforhealth.org.uk

Stephanie Tannis, East London and the City Mental Health NHS Trust

There are many organizations which offer support to people with mental health needs; mental health staff can help individuals to access this information. For example, an organization called Together; Working for Wellbeing (formerly called MACA) runs a range of mental health services across the country, engages in research and educates local communities about their own mental health needs.[13]

References

10 Alloway, R, Bebbington, P. The Buffer Theory of Social support – review of the literature. *Psychological Medicine* **17**: 91–108, 1987.

11 Simmons, S. Social Networks: their relevance to mental health nursing. *Journal of Advanced Nursing* **19**; 281–9, 1994.

12 Office of the Deputy Prime Minister. Mental Health and Social Exclusion: Social Exclusion Unit Report. ODPM: London, 2004.

13 See: www.together-uk.org

Supporting people with mental health needs in times of change

Many people feel threatened by change and may often respond with resistance. This is a natural coping strategy as change can be stressful, however, it is not always recognized as such. Change is not always negative: the anticipated losses must be weighed against the proposed advantages. Lewin in his classic theory of change (1958), describes the different stages of the change, process and how change is integrated into personal experience, implying that the change process itself is unpredictable. All life changes, whether negative or positive, carry a certain level of stress; mental health workers need to recognize and be able to support individuals who may be vulnerable to stress.

The role of the mental health nurse in managing change

- One of the most important aspects of supporting people through change is talking about it. Mental health workers should engage service users in discussing the change in their lives and actively listen to what it means for each individual.
- The mental health worker has an important role in information sharing and consultation with the service user, and can act as an information resource while supporting individuals to explore alternative options. It is important to give gradual exposure to information and change, allowing time for reflection and a review of feelings and goals.
- It is useful to engage in solution-focused discussions regarding change e.g. about the exact nature of the proposed change, what benefits may arise from this change for the individual or group and what the goal of this change will be. People can be encouraged to set realistic goals for themselves, and should be encouraged to accept that failure at various stages, or a change in a goal or plan is acceptable, and is part of the journey towards achieving what they want.
- It is important to express and acknowledge people's fears and anxieties about change; but the skilled mental health worker must be able to help them think about how negatives can be converted into positive outcomes.
- Mental health workers, family, friends, or support groups can provide the support and motivation needed at different stages of the change process.

Stephanie Tannis, East London and the City Mental Health NHS Trust

- Mental health services need to ensure that effective structures are in place to be able to respond to and support people through various life changes such as accommodation, relationship or social changes, or the loss of a loved one. Practical support may be required e.g. accessing social and financial support in a crisis.
- Mental health workers can help individuals develop and explore coping strategies, including accessing support groups in the community.

The essential key to helping individuals and families manage change is to ensure their involvement in each stage of the process, so that they have ownership of any decisions made.

The full version of the Mental Health National Occupational Standards is available at www.skillsforhealth.org.uk

Further reading

Lewin, K. The group reason and social change. In: E Macoby (ed.) *Readings in Social Psychology.* Holt, Reinhardt & Wilson; London, 1958.

Robinson, J. The role of resistance in the process of professional growth, Project 2000. *Journal of Advanced Nursing* **16**: 820, 1991.

Contributing to the management of risk and the protection of others

From the early 1990s, mental health service users have become more defined in terms of risk and dangerousness. This is despite the evidence that you are more likely to die at the hands of a member of your own family than be assaulted by somebody with a mental health problem. Alongside these beliefs, mental health policy has moved towards controlling those people considered a risk to others. For most mental health professionals, assessing and managing risk is now considered a key requirement of their practice with all age groups.

A press release from the Mental Health Foundation in October 2001 stated that risk could be reduced if all services supporting people with mental health problems used standard scales of assessment, shared information, and involved service users. Their report, 'Risk Management in Mental Health', suggested that many suicides and other incidents could have been avoided if those involved listened more carefully and shared information. For example:

- 24% of suicides were by people who had been in contact with mental health services in the year prior to death.
- Published inquiry reports reveal that incidents of violence committed by service users would have been less likely to occur had professionals listened to the family and others involved.

The use of risk assessment tools varies greatly across the country; and some form of standard is needed. As well as assessing risk, a holistic model should be used, including not only the service user's views on what risk they present at different times, but where risk occurs in other areas of their life. This could include racism, side-effects from medication, trauma, or separation from their family.

The culture of organizations should also be considered. This can influence the degree to which an individual or a team of professionals feel they have the organizational support to manage risk openly, or have to practice defensively.

Role of the mental health nurse

- Support the health and safety of yourself and individuals.
- Promote, monitor, and maintain health, safety and security in the working environment.
- Support individuals who are in distress.
- Contribute to protecting children and young people from danger, harm, and abuse.

Betsey Scott, East London and the City Mental Health NHS Trust

- Contribute to the protection of individuals from harm and abuse.
- Support individuals where abuse has been disclosed.
- Contribute to assessing and act upon risk of danger, harm, and abuse.
- Work with people to identify their needs for safety, support and engagement and how these needs can best be addressed.
- Enable people who are a risk to themselves and others to develop control.

The full version of the Mental Health National Occupational Standards is available at www.skillsforhealth.org.uk

Further reading

Langan, J, Lindow, V. Living with risk: mental health service user involvement in risk assessment and management. The Mental Health Foundation, Policy Press, 2001. London.

Nursing and Midwifery Council. Risk Management. NMC: London, 2000.

Ryan, T. Managing Crisis and Risk in Mental Health Nursing. Nelson Thornes: Cheltenham, 2004.

Addressing the mental health needs of the population

Public health is the science and art of preventing disease, prolonging life, and promoting health through the organized efforts of society. The public health agenda is concerned with improving the health of the population, rather than treating the diseases of individual patients.

Positive mental health attributes of a population include:
- Feeling satisfied, optimistic, and hopeful.
- Being confident and hopeful in all aspects of life.
- Having a relaxed and enthusiastic attitude.
- Being interested in other people and the community you live in.

Poor mental health is associated with:
- Increased risk of poor physical health.
- Poor self management of chronic illness.
- Health damaging behaviours such as smoking, substance misuse, unwanted pregnancy, and poor diet.

There are links between despair, anger, frustration, hopelessness, poor self-worth, and higher cholesterol levels, hypertension, and susceptibility to infection (these are high risk factors for coronary heart disease and stroke).

Mental health problems cost approximately £77 billion per year in terms of economic losses and premature death, with approximately 900,000 people claiming incapacity benefit for a mental health problem.[14]

Mental illness prevalence rates are not an indicator of the mental health of a nation as many mental illness are undetected e.g. depression in the elderly.

The mental health of a population cannot be addressed in isolation from the broader community perspective. A range of other factors are involved that are addressed by national and local polices including, mental health promotion, violence and abuse (feeling safe in the community), equality and inclusion (access to services), early years care, life long learning, employment (healthy work places), later life, and community regeneration. All these have a bearing on the positive mental health attributes of a population and are addressed thorough local council policies.

Public Health in England has seven core functions, all of which can be applied to mental health:
- Health surveillance, monitoring, and analysis.
- Investigation of disease outbreaks, epidemics, and risk to health.
- Establishing, designing, and managing health promotion and disease prevention programmes.
- Enabling and empowering communities to promote health and reduce inequalities.
- Creating and sustaining cross-government (national and local) partnerships to improve health and reduce inequalities.

Betsey Scott, East London and the City Mental Health NHS Trust

- Ensuring compliance with regulations and laws to protect and promote health.
- Developing and maintaining a well-educated and trained, multi-disciplinary public health workforce.

Role of the mental health nurse

- To keep an open mind.
- Be alert to areas where mental health needs may be changing.
- Report where current means of meeting needs are failing to serve the requirements of some section of the population, e.g. interpretation services.
- Ensure equity of provision and access to all.
- Understand that 'population' may refer to a local or geographical area or a group of people with specific needs.

The full version of the Mental Health National Occupational Standards is available at www.skillsforhealth.org.uk

Reference

14 Sainsbury's Centre for Mental Health. SCMH: London, 2003.

Further reading

Levin, BC, Petrila, J *Mental Health Services: a public health perspective*. Oxford University Press: New York, 2004.

Working with groups and communities to address their mental health needs

The Department of Health's National Service Framework for Mental Health gives a high priority to the mental health needs of groups and communities.[15] This framework set out a programme of modernization and reform of mental health services, with a view to providing consistent high quality services. The framework's standards cover all aspects of mental health care, and firmly indicate that partnership between health and social services is essential for successful implementation.

Individuals may become socially excluded as a consequence or cause of the experience of mental illness and the National Service Framework seeks to address this in its first standard. It states that health and social services should combat discrimination against individuals and groups with mental health problems, and promote their social inclusion. The government has put in place policies and initiatives to support the National Service Framework and promote social inclusion. Most notably, the Social Exclusion Unit was created in 1997 to make recommendations to tackle exclusion on a practice level. 📖 Social inclusion.

The role of the mental health nurse and service provision

There are many ways that professionals can work with local groups and communities:

- The professional can work in partnership with, and be a resource to statutory and voluntary agencies and service users, with their role and agenda being determined by the needs of the community. The mental health needs of individuals and families experiencing mental health difficulties must be at the heart of service provision.
- Mental health services must engage with and include service users and carers in the planning, implementation and review of projects, new services and community initiatives. Mental health workers should support service users to become involved in the planning and implementation of local projects, mental health services and national initiatives, acting as a voice for mental health service users, to ensure that their views are heard and interests considered. Stephanie Tannis
- Mental health organizations must consult and involve local community groups in the planning and provision of mental health services, to ensure that needs are correctly identified and that services are culturally appropriate for that particular community.
- Links can be formed with schools, resident's associations, public sector services such as the police, religious groups, and local businesses to open up communication between the wider community and service users as part of promoting social inclusion. Mental health professionals are well positioned to offer to sit on local committees.

Stephanie Tannis, East London and the City Mental Health NHS Trust

- The positive promotion of mental health services within the community can bridge the gap between knowledge and understanding of mental health issues, and the myths that may abound. It is important for mental health professionals to give information using a range of methods for example, public education programmes and forging links with non-English speaking communities, making efforts to provide information in different languages.

Effective collaboration with community groups includes ensuring that mental health services reflect the community they serve, e.g. by recruiting staff from the community. Mental health organizations have a responsibility to provide specific training such as cultural competence and public health awareness for its workforce.

The full version of the Mental Health National Occupational Standards is available at www.skillsforhealth.org.uk

Reference

15 Department of Health. A National Service Framework for Mental Health. DOH: London, 1999.

Influencing organizations' behaviour and services so as to promote people's mental health

Influencing at an organizational level is the role of senior management for service planning and development, by identifying areas where community networks and partnerships could inform and support practice, by bringing together relevant people and organizations to be involved, enabling practitioners and agencies to work collaboratively to improve mental health. However, all mental health practitioners have the opportunity to influence organizations through the implementation of multi-agency care planning (CPA).

Role of the mental health nurse

- Contribute to the development, maintenance, and evaluation of systems to promote the rights, responsibilities, equality, and diversity of individuals.
- Contribute to promoting a culture that values and respects the diversity of individuals.
- Assess how environments and practices can be maintained and improved to promote mental health.
- Encourage and develop action plans to enable others to see the value of improving environments and practices to promote mental health.
- Raise awareness of the value of employment, training, and education for people with mental health needs.
- Negotiate and agree placements to offer to people with mental health needs opportunities in employment, training, and education.
- Support employers and others in their work with individuals with mental health needs.
- Raise awareness of the housing needs of people with mental health needs.
- Raise awareness of the value of leisure activities for people with mental health needs.

The full version of the Mental Health National Occupational Standards is available at www.skillsforhealth.org.uk

The Mental Health Foundation states that over 25 million people in the United Kingdom spend a large part of their lives at work. For those in the population with a mental health problem, work is an important coping mechanism. It not only gives people financial security – the ability to pay a mortgage and pension contributions for example – but it also provides a sense of purpose and value, preventing the social exclusion that many service users suffer. However, only 17% of people with a diagnosis of serious mental illness are economically active.[16]

Betsy Scott, East London and the City Mental Health NHS Trust

The ability to influence organizations to be more proactive in supporting their employees with mental health issues already exists to some degree. However, government legislation will require organizations to pay more than lip service to supporting service users in employment. The right to work is enshrined in Article 23 of the United Nations Declaration of Human Rights, which states that 'everyone has a right to work, to free choice of employment, to just and favourable conditions of work and to protection against unemployment'.[17]

To achieve this aim, assisting service users to gain and sustain employment should be considered an important 'treatment' in its own right. Having service users in employment is central to achieving many of the targets for mental health services, which have been set over the last decade. For example the Health of the Nation Targets and the Mental Health National Service Framework.[18,19]

References

16 Office for National Statistics: 1982–3. www.statistics.gov.uk.
17 United Nations. Declaration of Human Rights, Article 23. www.un.org/overview/rights.
18 Department of Health. Health of the Nation Targets. DoH: London, 1992.
19 Department of Health. A National Service Framework for Mental Health. DOH: London, 1999.

Further reading

Deponte, P. *Pull yourself together: a survey of the stigma and discrimination faced by people who experience mental distress*: 2000. Mental Health Foundation London.
Faulkner, A, Layzell, S. Strategies for Living.: 2000. Mental Health foundation London.
Dunns. Creating accepting communities. *Journal of Medical Ethics* 2002; 28:58–59.

Influencing the way in which organizations interact to benefit mental health services

In the UK, mental health problems are a leading cause of distress, illness, and disability, and they carry a considerable financial cost for organizations. The Mental Health Foundation estimates that 80 million working days are lost every year in the UK due to mental illness, and that the cost to employers is £1.2 billion. Despite this, it is not easy to identify companies who are proactive in supporting mental health issues within their own infrastructure, or who are prepared to work collaboratively to benefit mental health service users.

Role of the mental health nurse

- Sustain and review collaborative working.
- Work with and through community networks and partnerships.
- Explore, initiate, and develop collaborative working relationships.
- Develop and sustain effective working relationships with staff in other agencies.
- Work with others to facilitate the transfer of individuals between agencies or services.
- Lead the development of inter-agency services for addressing mental health needs.
- Lead the implementation of inter-agency services for addressing mental health needs.
- Monitor, evaluate, and improve inter-agency services for addressing mental health needs.

The full version of the Mental Health National Occupational Standards is available at www.skillsforhealth.org.uk

Influencing the work place

A report from the Mental Health Foundation called 'Out at Work' made the following recommendations to support organizations to change:

- The Disability Rights Commission should give priority to addressing discrimination in relation to people with mental health problems.
- The government needs to recognize the importance of employment for people with mental health problems and implement initiatives that promote, support and, where necessary, provide opportunities for returning to employment.
- The government and all agencies working in mental health should consider a campaign encouraging people to 'come out' about their mental health problems, so it is not seen as a minority issue.
- The benefits system should be re-examined so it does not penalize those who return to work, and then find they are not well enough and have to leave.

Betsey Scott, East London and the City Mental Health NHS Trust

- Employers should audit their workplace, identify elements of practice or culture that may be detrimental to mental health, and seek to address these.
- Employers should consider policies such as a gradual return to work after a period of mental illness in order to support and retain valued employees.
- Employers should consider giving time off work for counselling or psychotherapy appointments as they would for other medical appointments.
- There should be mental health awareness training in schools to ensure that future employees and colleagues have a better understanding of mental health problems, and of how to look after their own well-being.

Further reading

The Mental Health Foundation. Mental Health in the Workplace. MHF: London, 1999.
OPCS surveys of psychiatry morbidity in Great Britain, Report 5. The Stationery Office: London.
Singleton N, Bumpstead R, O'Brein M, Lee A, Meltzer H. Psychiatric Morbidity among adults living in private households. International Review of Psychiatry 2003; **15**:65–73 Routledge.

Influencing the way in which others recognize and respond to people with mental health needs

Discriminatory attitudes pervade our media, and a lack of knowledge can often lead to unrealistic fears and prejudices against those with mental health problems. It is important to consider our own actions in order to influence the way that others respond to people with mental health problems. Promote the rights, responsibilities, equality, and diversity of individuals.

The mental health professional can help by:

- Acting in such a way as to ensure that the rights of people with mental health needs are respected, and that they are treated within an environment of equality and transparency. Dignity and privacy should always be paramount, and choice should be given where possible.
- Always acting within the law and in accordance with Human Rights legislation. Particular attention needs to be given to communication which reflects the above, and refrains from the use of vulgar or discriminatory terms for those with mental health problems.
- Raising positive awareness of mental health issues, through educating fellow non-mental health professionals in primary, secondary and tertiary care. Other organizations can be targeted such as social service colleagues, schools, and colleges.
- Contributing to developing, maintaining and evaluation of systems that respect the rights and interests of individuals, to ensure that everyone is treated equally and that promote confidence in you and your organization.

Information and advice on promoting positive attitudes can be obtained via the following websites:

- Mind's Fact sheet – 'Public Attitude to Mental Distress'[20]
- Department of Health publication – 'Attitudes to Mental Illness'[21]
- Mental Health Media Council – 'Anti discriminatory toolkit'[22]

Role of the mental health nurse

- Take responsibility for your own continuing professional development.
- Represent the organization in courts and formal hearings e.g. mental health review tribunals.
- Contribute to raising awareness of mental health issues.
- Promote the equality, diversity, rights, and responsibilities of individuals.
- Promote the needs, rights, interests, and responsibilities of individuals within the community.

Johanna Turner, Performance Panel Coordinator and Legal Advisor, Newham PCT, London

- Assess the need for, and plan awareness raising of mental health issues e.g. in schools.
- Support the implementation, monitoring, evaluation, and improvement of awareness raising around mental health issues e.g. world mental health day.
- Support others in understanding people's mental health needs and how these can be addressed in their work.
- Support and challenge other workers on specific aspects of their practice.

The full version of the Mental Health National Occupational Standards is available at www.skillsforhealth.org.uk

References

20 www.mind.org.uk/Information/Factsheets/Public+attitudes/
21 www.dh.gov.uk/PublicationsAndStatistics/Publications/PublicationsPolicyAndGuidance/ Publications PolicyAndGuidanceArticle/fs/en?CONTENT_ID=4074810&chk=4nmfbo
22 www.mhmedia.com/products/new.html

Essential Shared Capabilities

The Essential Shared Capabilities (ESC) for mental health practice

The ESCs are a set of statements that outline the capabilities thought to be essential for delivery of effective mental health care. They were developed by a representative group of people working in, receiving, and having an interest in mental health, including service users and carers. They are designed for use by all mental health practitioners.

Capability	Meaning
Working in partnership	Working actively with users, carers, families, colleagues, lay people and other agencies. Managing conflict.
Respecting diversity	Working with people in manner that respects and values diversity in relation to age, race, culture, disability, gender, spirituality, and sexuality.
Practising ethically	Recognizing rights, acknowledging power differentials and minimizing them. Being accountable to users and carers and adhering to professional, legal, and local codes of practice.
Challenging inequality	Working with the causes and consequences of stigma, discrimination, social exclusion, and inequality. Developing and sustaining the valued social roles of people.
Promoting recovery	Helping users and carers develop hope and optimism, so that they may live without incapacitating mental health problems.
Identifying people's needs and strengths	Agreeing with users and carers their health and social needs within their chosen lifestyles.
Providing service user-centred care	Agreeing achievable and meaningful goals from the user and carers' perspectives, implementing actions to meet these goals and evaluating the outcomes.
Making a difference	Contributing to the delivery of evidence and values-based care.
Promoting safety and positive risk-taking	Enabling people to help decide the level of risk they want to take with their health and safety.
Personal development and learning	Participating in professional and personal development through supervision, appraisal and reflective practice, life-long learning and keeping up-to-date with changes in practice.

Peter Lindley, Sainsbury Centre for Mental Health

Further reading

Department of Health. The Ten Essential Shared Capabilities for Mental Health Practice. DoH: London, 2004.

Working in partnership

The first of the Ten Essential Shared Capabilities (ESC) is Working in Partnership

Partnerships are the key to success!

Although all of the ESC are interrelated working in partnership is the foundation of all the care and treatment provided by all mental health practitioners. It is critical to the success of everything that we do, for and on behalf of the people we serve. Indeed without harmonious partnerships with service users and colleagues there are serious doubts about the extent to which it is possible to demonstrate any of the other ESC.

You might find it interesting to reflect on the following question: Is it possible to demonstrate the other ESCs such as 'Respecting Diversity', or 'Promoting Recovery', without working in partnership?

What does this capability involve?

- A commitment to respecting people who rely on our services – service users, carers, and families as active partners with contributions and choices to make, **NOT** passive recipients of care.
- Respectful engagement and participation of everyone involved in receiving or providing mental health care. At every stage and level of the services provided.
- Actively sustaining these relationships and bringing them to an appropriate conclusion when their contribution has achieved the desired results.

What can you do to develop this capability?

- Learn what life is like for the people we serve. What is their lived experience of mental distress and what impact does this have on their willingness to engage with the services we provide?
- Learn about the roles and responsibilities of the different practitioners who provide mental health care in both the statutory and independent sector.
- Develop a clear account of your and other practitioners' roles, responsibilities, and limitations.
- Make a commitment to regular appraisal and supervision to ensure that you review and update your communication skills.
- Learn from working alongside the people you serve and make sure that you routinely ask them for feedback.
- Learn from your peers and colleagues-particularly the people whose practise you admire. What is that they do that might help you to become a capable practitioner?

Peter Lindley, Sainsbury Centre for Mental Health

Conclusion

Developing the capability to work in partnership is fundamental to your effectiveness as a practitioner. You should make a lasting commitment to reviewing your knowledge and abilities throughout your career. The people you serve and inspirational colleagues can provide you with valuable feedback and important role models.

Further reading

Edwards, K. *Partnership working in mental health care: the nursing dimension.* Elsevier: London, 2005.

Rose, D. Users Voices; the perspectives of Mental Health Service Users on Community and Hospital care. SCMH: London. Download the extract free from www.scmh.org.uk

Sainsbury's Centre for Mental Health. Taking Your Partners Using Opportunities for Inter-Agency Partnership in Mental Health. SCMH: London, 2000. Download the Briefing Paper free from www.scmh.org.uk

Respecting diversity

The second of the ESC is Respecting Diversity and this is defined as:

Respecting diversity – we could do a lot better

We are fortunate to be practising at a time when our society is composed of a wonderfully vibrant and diverse population of peoples of all ages, backgrounds, talents, and cultures. However, it is clear that mental health services do not always respond positively to this extraordinarily rich variety of peoples. They fail to take account of the unique identities and needs of many people from ethnic or other minority backgrounds. Recent reports are particularly critical of service failures in relation to young African-Caribbean men and women.[1,2]

What does this capability involve?

- A commitment to challenging existing values and attitudes about age, race, culture, disability, gender, spirituality, and sexuality can be examined and challenged.
- Promoting systems, structures, policies, and therapeutic interventions that value, respect, and acknowledge the positive contributions of people from diverse backgrounds.

What can you do to develop this capability?

- Learn about the lives of the people we serve and their experience of mental distress and discrimination, particularly the interaction of their distress with their age, gender, race, culture, disability, spirituality, and sexuality.
- Find out what local people at risk of discrimination feel about local services.
- Build alliances with the community groups and organizations that represent and support people at risk of discrimination.
- Examine your practise (with your supervisor) to ascertain to what extent it demonstrates your commitment to equal opportunities for all the people you serve.

Conclusion

We live in a time of wonderful cultural diversity in which mental health practitioners are faced with significant challenges. They need to make their practice much more responsive to differences in age, sexuality, spirituality, gender, and ethnicity.

📖 Culturally capable mental health nursing
📖 Working with people from different cultural and ethnic groups

Peter Lindley, Sainsbury Centre for Mental Health

References

1 Sainsbury Centre for Mental Health. Breaking the Circles of Fear: a review of the relationship between mental health services and African and Caribbean Communities. SCMH: London, 2002.
2 Department of Health. Delivering Race Equality: A framework for action, Mental Health Services Consultation Document. DoH: London, 2005.

Further reading

Fernando, S. *Cultural Diversity, mental health and psychiatry: the struggle against racisim*. Brunner-Routledge: London, 2003.

Practising ethically

Practising ethically involves recognizing rights and acknowledging power differentials and minimizing them. It also means being accountable to users and carers, and adhering to professional, legal and local codes of practice[3].

In order to practise ethically, the mental health nurse will:
- Uphold the legal and human rights of service users.
- Identify the networks that support the service user and facilitate the contribution of significant others in the users' care, if they agree.
- Work with all people in an ethical, honest, and non-judgemental manner.
- Enable the user to make choices and to participate in care and treatment.
- Practice in a legally and ethically accountable manner, and in a way that their care can be scrutinized by others.
- Uphold users and carers' rights and responsibilities; maintain their privacy, dignity, and safety using the principle of informed consent.
- Work as a member of the care team in maintaining a safe environment that prevents and manages violence in a therapeutic manner.
- Adhere to the NMC Code of Professional Conduct.
- Adhere to the Mental Health Act, Code of Practice, and the Mental Capacity Bill.
- Work within the boundaries of local complaints and management systems.

Peter Lindley, Sainsbury Centre for Mental Health

Reference

3 Department of Health. The Ten Essential Shared Capabilities for Mental Health Practice. DoH: London, 2004.

Challenging inequality

The 'wounds' of inequality

Many people with mental health problems will also have to contend with the effects of widespread stigma, discrimination, and inequality. The negative consequences of this discrimination occur accross every aspect of their lives. These 'wounds' are deeply distressing and can have a profoundly negative impact on their mental health status and their potential to take control of their recovery to lead a full and satisfying life.

The 'wounds' include (Wolfensberger, 1992):

- Low social status/feeling not part of society.
- Rejection by family, friends, and communities.
- Loss of relationships.
- Loss of choice and control over their lives.
- At risk of neglect and abuse.
- Poverty.
- Poor physical health, health care requirements overlooked.

Recent surveys indicate that people with mental health problems are amongst the most discriminated groups in our society (MIND, 1999).

What does this capability involve?

- A commitment to keeping up to date with the latest knowledge about the nature and consequences of stigma and discrimination.
- Applying this knowledge in practise through interventions that are directed not only at assisting the person and their families and friends to resolve mental distress, but are also clearly directed at actively challenging and overcoming the 'wounds' of inequality.
- Developing alliances with community groups, advocates and generic services able to provide some of the supports people may need to overcome the 'wounds' and develop valued social roles.
- Supporting activists and campaigns aimed at challenging the conditions that allow inequality to thrive.

What can you do to develop this capability?

- Learn from the people and the communities that you serve about the inequalitities that they experience; ask them about the impact inequality has on their lives.
- Find out the extent to which mental health services amplify inequalities and make a commitment to working with others to make positive changes in this.
- Develop skills in person-centred planning and use these to provide care that actively and specifically seeks to help people develop valued social roles and remove the inequalities they experience.
- Join a network of like-minded people keen to improve their knowledge and practice.

Peter Lindley, Sainsbury Centre for Mental Health

Conclusion

People with mental health problems are often the victims of discrimination and inequality. Most of the care that they receive fails to take account of this and sometimes adds to it. Mental health practitioners need to focus more clearly on developing their capabilities to challenge inequality through their practise and in alliance with community groups and advocates.

📖 Culturally capable mental health nursing
📖 Working with people from different cultural and ethnic groups

Further reading

MIND. Not Just Sticks and Stones. MIND: London, 1999.
Pilgrim, D, Rogers, A. *Mental Health and Inequality*. London Palgrave Macmillan: 2002.
Wolfensberger, W. A Brief Introduction to Social Role Valorisation as a higher order concept for structuring human services. Training Institute for Human Service Planning: Syracuse NY, 1992.

Promoting recovery

Promoting recovery involves helping users and carers develop hope and optimism so that they may begin to live without incapacitating mental health problems[4].

In order to promote recovery, the mental health nurse will:
- Understand that the process of recovery is unique to each person.
- Understand the role of hope in recovery.
- Accept that recovery does not always mean the elimination or curing of symptoms.
- Understand that the service user's needs should determine the planning and delivery of support.
- Be responsive and flexible to the user's needs.
- Present positive views of people who experience mental health distress.
- Work with advocacy groups in upholding the rights and interests of users.
- Enable the user to participate in community activities.

Peter Lindley, Sainsbury Centre for Mental Health

Reference

4 Department of Health. The Ten Essential Shared Capabilities for Mental Health Practice. DoH: London, 2004.

Identifying people's needs and strengths

Identifying people's needs and strengths involves agreeing with users and carers on their health and social needs, within their chosen lifestyles.

In order to identify people's strengths and weaknesses, the mental health nurse will:

- Gather information from a range of sources e.g. the person, significant others, other disciplines, and agencies.
- Conduct an holistic assessment focusing on the strengths and needs of individual users and carers.
- Identify the personal, social, cultural, and spiritual strengths and weaknesses of the user.
- Promote the physical and mental health of the user, and understand how these elements impact upon each other, and on other parts of the system.
- Understand how other parts of the person's health system impact upon the physical and mental health of the user.

Peter Lindley, Sainsbury Centre for Mental Health

Reference
5 Department of Health. The Ten Essential Shared Capabilities for Mental Health Practice. DoH: London, 2004.

Providing service user-centred care

Providing service user-centred care involves agreeing achievable and meaningful goals from both the user and the carers' perspectives, implementing actions to meet these goals, and evaluating the outcomes[6].

In order to provide service user-centred care, the mental health nurse will:

- Work in partnership with the user to help them describe their goals in a precise and meaningful manner.
- Enable the user to identify and use their strengths to achieve their goals and aspirations.
- Incorporate the resources from the user's support network into nursing care.
- Develop agreed goals based on the user's needs.
- Set SMART goals i.e. goals that are Specific, Measurable, Achievable, Realistic, and Time-Oriented.

Understand the difference between short and long-term goals.

Peter Lindley, Sainsbury Centre for Mental Health

Reference

6 Department of Health. The Ten Essential Shared Capabilities for Mental Health Practice. DoH: London, 2004.

Making a difference

Making a difference involves contributing to the delivery of evidence and values-based care[7].

In order to make a difference to the care of users and their significant others, the mental health nurse will:

- Identify the impact of any problem on the life of the service user and their significant others.
- Have a working knowledge of evidence-based interventions and values-based practice.
- Use best practice and clinical guidelines such as those published by NICE.
- Practise according to the best available evidence.
- Work with other professionals and agencies in delivering care based on the best available evidence.
- Work in partnership with users and their significant others in delivering care based on the best available evidence.

Peter Lindley, Sainsbury Centre for Mental Health

Reference

7 Department of Health. The Ten Essential Shared Capabilities for Mental Health Practice. DoH: London, 2004.

Promoting safety and positive risk-taking

Promoting safety and positive risk-taking involves enabling people to help decide the level of risk they want to take with their health and safety[8].

In order to promote safety and positive risk taking, the mental health nurse will:

- Work in partnership with users and carers, especially those who do not engage with services.
- Understand factors associated with the risk of self-harm or harm to others.
- Educate users and carers about the limitations of services in promoting safety and managing risk.
- Conduct and contribute to effective risk assessments, identifying the risk to the person and others.
- Implement and contribute to the implementation of risk management programmes involving users and their carers and other agencies.
- Minimize identified risks.
- Work within national and local policies and procedures for reducing and managing users' risk to self and others.
- Understand the CPA and contribute to the CPA in ensuring safe and effective care.
- Have a working knowledge of the role of other agencies in managing and reducing risk.
- Use, and contribute to the use of psychosocial interventions by others in managing and reducing risk.

Peter Lindley, Sainsbury Centre for Mental Health

Reference

8 Department of Health. The Ten Essential Shared Capabilities for Mental Health Practice. DoH: London, 2004.

Personal development and learning

Personal development and learning involves participating in professional and personal development through supervision, appraisal, and reflective practice, life-long learning, and keeping up-to-date with changes in practice[9].

In order to meet his or her own personal development and learning the mental health nurse will:

- Access education and training based on the best available evidence.
- Have a development plan outlining their hopes, aspirations, and plans, that is reviewed annually.
- Recognize the importance of their employer in helping them meet their personal and professional goals.
- Acknowledge their own responsibilities for meeting their personal and professional goals.
- Set personal and professional goals that are achievable.
- Use supervision, and reflect upon their practice regularly.
- Seek opportunities for supervision and personal and professional development.

Peter Lindley, Sainsbury Centre for Mental Health

Reference

9 Department of Health The Ten Essential Shared Capabilities for Mental Health Practice. DoH: London, 2004.

Index

Mental Health (Care and Treatment) (Scotland) Act 2003

Section/Part	Duration	Mental Health Commision/ Mental Health Tribunal	Appeal	Consent
36 Emergency detention in hospital	72 hours	MWC informed if MHO consent not obtained	No Can be revoked by Approved Medical Practitioner	MHO, where practicable
44 Short-term detention in hospital	28 days Can be extended by 3 days prior to CTO	MWC/MHT to be informed within 7 days	Patient/named person can apply to Tribunal for revocation of certificate	MHO Named person to be informed
299 Nurse's holding power	2 hours Can be extended by 1 hour to allow examination to be carried out	MWC to be informed in writing	No	No
Part 7 Compulsory Treatment Order Treatment enforced either in hospital or community setting	6 months, followed by 6 months, then 12 monthly	Tribunal makes decision on application	At time of Tribunal hearing and After 3 months	No